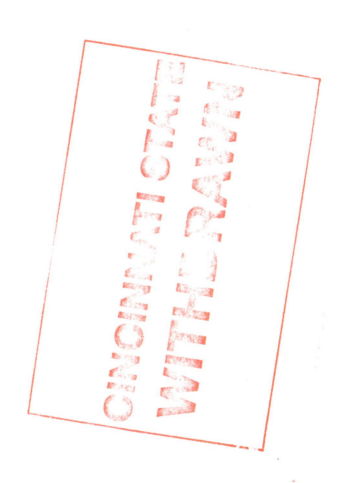

Rapid Interpretation of Ventilator Waveforms

Second Edition

Jonathan B. Waugh, Ph.D., RRT, RPFT
University of Alabama Birmingham
Critical Care Department
Birmingham, Alabama

Vijay M. Deshpande, M.S., RRT, FAARC
Georgia State University
Division of Respiratory Therapy
Atlanta, Georgia

Melissa K. Brown, BSRT, RRT-NPS
Grossmont Community College
Health Sciences Department
El Cajon, California
and
Sharp Memorial Hospital
Pulmonary Department
San Diego, CA

Robert J. Harwood, M.S.A., RRT-NPS
Georgia State University
Division of Respiratory Therapy
Atlanta, Georgia

PEARSON

Prentice
Hall   Upper Saddle River, New Jersey 07458

Publisher: Julie Levin Alexander
Assistant to Publisher: Regina Bruno
Executive Editor: Mark Cohen
Editorial Assistant: Nicole Ragonese
Director of Production and Manufacturing: Bruce Johnson
Managing Production Editor: Patrick Walsh
Manufacturing Buyer: Pat Brown
Senior Design Coordinator: Maria Guglielmo
Composition and Page Layout: Linda D. Waugh, Graphic Illustrator
Director of Marketing: Karen Allman
Marketing Manager: Harper Coles
Marketing Coordinator: Michael Sirinides
Marketing Assistant: Patricia Linard
Copy Editor: Donna Cullen-Dolce
Cover Design: Gary Sella
Cover Illustration: Courtesy of Advanced Body Scan, Newport Beach, CA
Printer/Binder: R.R. Donnelley & Sons
Cover Printer: Phoenix Color Corporation

Pearson Education LTD.
Pearson Education Australia PTY, Limited
Pearson Education Singapore, Pte. Ltd
Pearson Education North Asia Ltd
Pearson Education Canada, Ltd.
Pearson Educación de Mexico, S.A. de C.V.
Pearson Education -- Japan
Pearson Education Malaysia, Pte. Ltd
Pearson Education, Incorporated, Upper Saddle River, New Jersey

10 9 8 7 6 5 4 3 2
ISBN 0-13-174922-6

Right Mainstem Intubation F-V and P-V Loops, 129
Progression to Extubation Scalars, 130
Turbulent Baseline Flow Rate Scalars, 131
High Frequency Ventilation, 132

CONTENTS

PREFACE

This text introduces ventilator waveforms. It is intended to serve as a complement to a mechanical ventilation textbook and as a reference convenient to carry in the clinical setting.

The first chapter provides clear, easy-to-read conceptual illustrations to aid in comprehension. Examples of real waveforms are provided next to the conceptual renderings to allow the learner to become comfortable with viewing waveforms with normal artifact present. The subsequent chapters utilize mostly real recordings of ventilator waveforms.

The rationale behind the format of this text is to provide a simple, portable reference and workbook that can be used at the bedside as well as the classroom. Descriptions and commentary are kept to a minimum to enhance clarity and readability. Ventilator waveform topics that are experimental, in limited use, or not considered mainstream are given little attention in keeping with this book's introductory theme.

It would be impractical and ponderous to attempt to include all possible examples of ventilator waveforms that can be seen in the clinical setting. The goal of this book is to impart an understanding of how waveforms are generated, which will allow the practitioner to deduce the cause and implications of previously unseen as well as familiar waveforms. Understanding waveforms, instead of memorizing many patterns, aids in problem solving and correction of abnormal conditions and prepares clinicians to adapt to future yet unknown modes of ventilation.

REVIEWERS

Robert Tralongo, MBA, RRT-NPS
Respiratory Therapy Program
Molloy College
Rockville Center, New York

Stanley M. Pearson, MSEd, RRT
Respiratory Therapy Program
SIUC/School of Allied Health
Carbondale, Illinois

Heidi Story, AS, RRT, RCP
Respiratory Therapy Program
Ohlone College
Fremont, California

Susan Pilbeam, MS, RRT, FAARC
Respiratory Care Educational Consultant
St. Augustine, Florida

Case studies to accompany this book may be reviewed at www.prenhall.com/waugh

FOREWORD

Change is a fact of life. It is the first and most important indicator of progress. The profession of Respiratory Care has clearly changed and progressed over time. It is amazing for me to reflect on my early days as an "oxygen technician" and contemplate the four decades of change in the profession that I have witnessed. In the mid 1960s ventilators were simple pneumatic or electrically operated machines and the only modes of ventilation provided were assist, assist/control or control. Few of the ventilators available in the 1960s included any type of monitor or alarm. Today, revolutionary changes in mechanical ventilation have occurred; the ventilators are controlled by multiple levels of microprocessors. They can deliver a large variety of both pressure-targeted and volume-targeted modes of ventilation. They have incorporated what seems like an unlimited number of alarms. Some units including over 300 potential error codes identifying malfunctions. Most importantly this current generation of ICU ventilators provides detailed patient monitoring. Almost every one of the ICU ventilators on the market today displays waveforms of pressure, flow, and volume as well as pressure-volume and flow-volume loops. However, the dilemma facing many practitioners is a desire to use this data but a lack of appropriately packaged materials to help them interpret the information presented in these waveforms.

This textbook by Waugh, Deshpande, Brown, and Harwood solves this dilemma. Its presentation of waveform interpretation is a welcome and needed addition to the Respiratory Care literature. In this textbook these authors present the basic information needed by every practitioner to be able to interpret ventilation waveforms. This textbook provides a clear and concise guide to understanding and appreciation of the information present in the waveforms depicted on ICU ventilators. The authors state that the goal of this textbook is "to import an understanding of how waveforms are generated which will allow the practitioner to deduce the cause and implications of previously unseen as well as familiar waveforms." These authors have achieved their goal! The information in this textbook is presented in a manner that is easy to understand and most importantly for this topic is presented with the use of numerous illustrations and examples. This is an excellent textbook for both students and seasoned clinicians and should be a welcomed addition to the library of all respiratory care practitioners.

We have clearly come a long way as a profession; the need to understand the information in this textbook is critical for today's respiratory therapists. I cannot even imagine that we would have been ready for such a book back in the 1960s and 1970s.

Robert M. Kacmarek, Ph.D., RRT, FAARC
Professor of Anesthesiology, Harvard Medical School
Director, Respiratory Care
Massachusetts General Hospital
Boston, Massachusetts

CHAPTER 1
VENTILATOR GRAPHICS AND CLINICAL APPLICATIONS

BASIC CONCEPTS

Four basic parameters are most descriptive of mechanical ventilation: pressure, volume, flow, and time. Conventionally, these parameters are plotted against each other to reflect changes associated with changes in pathology. Normally, three graphs, called scalars comprising of flow vs. time, volume vs. time, and pressure vs. time are used. Other graphs such as flow-volume loop and pressure-volume loop provide quick information on certain changes in lung function. In order to be consistent in initial parameters, the following example will serve as a baseline and a reference point to compare any variations in the settings or in lung functions.

CLINICAL EXAMPLE The following example is designed to demonstrate to the reader how the computerized graphic system incorporated in the ventilators actually draws these waveforms based on the set parameters and calculated parameters. The example provides illustrations of effects of changes in ventilator modes on the tracings of pressure, volume, and flow plotted against time.

A post–open heart patient is brought in the intensive care unit and placed on a volume ventilator on the following parameters:

Tidal Volume (V_T)	750 mL or 0.75 L
Respiratory Frequency (f)	15 breath/min or respiratory cycles/min
Inspiratory Flow Rate ($\dot{V}$)	30 L/min
Airways Resistance (R_{AW})	10 cm H_2O/L/sec
Respiratory System Compliance (C_{RS})	0.05 L/cm H_2O or 50 mL/cm H_2O
Mode	Control

EFFECT OF FLOW RATE ON INSPIRATORY AND EXPIRATORY TIME

Increased inspiratory flow rate (Figure 1-2) decreases inspiratory time and allows for a longer expiration time, conversely if the flow rate is decreased, the inspiratory time increases and the expiratory time decreases.

The inspiratory time can be calculated by dividing the delivered tidal volume by the inspiratory flow rate (mL/sec). For the initial settings, V_T = 750 mL, f = 15 cycles/min, $\dot{V}$ = 30 L/min, T_C = 4 sec, T_I = 1.5 seconds, T_E = 2.5 seconds, and inspiratory flow rate = 30 L/min = 30 L/60 sec = 0.5 L/sec = 500 mL/sec.

$$T_I = \frac{\text{tidal volume}}{\text{flow rate}}$$

$$T_I = \frac{\text{tidal volume}}{\text{flow rate}} = \frac{750 \text{ mL}}{500 \text{ mL/sec}} = 1.5 \text{ sec}$$

Observe Figure 1-2A. The graphic indicates the effect of increasing flow rate from 30 L/min to 60 L/min. Notice that the inspiratory time decreased from 1.5 seconds to 0.75 seconds and the expiratory time increased from 2.5 seconds to 3.25 seconds. Recognize that the cycle time remained 4 seconds. If the flow rate is doubled from 30 L/min to 60 L/min, the inspiratory time decreases by half, from 1.5 seconds to 0.75 seconds, thus allowing for a longer expiratory time (3.25 seconds).

$$T_I = \frac{\text{tidal volume}}{\text{flow rate}} = \frac{750 \text{ mL}}{1000 \text{ mL/sec}} = 0.75 \text{ sec}$$

As shown in Figure 1-2B, if the inspiratory flow rate is decreased, the inspiratory time increases. This is shown in Figure 1-2B. The inspiratory flow rate is decreased from 30 L/min to 22.5 L/min (22.5 L/min = 22.5 L/60 sec = 0.375 L/sec = 375 mL/sec). The change in flow rate increases the inspiratory time from 1.5 seconds to 2.0 seconds, which in turn decreases the expiratory time from 2.5 seconds to 2.0 seconds.

$$T_I = \frac{\text{tidal volume}}{\text{flow rate}} = \frac{750 \text{ mL}}{375 \text{ mL/sec}} = 2.0 \text{ sec}$$

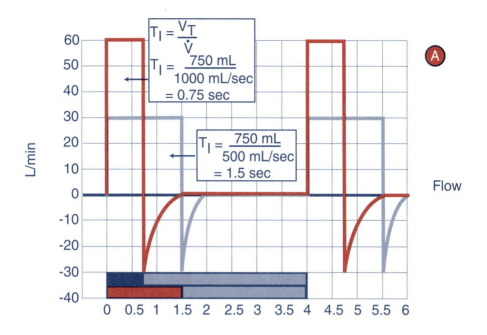

$$T_I = \frac{V_T}{\dot{V}}$$

$$T_I = \frac{750\ mL}{1000\ mL/sec} = 0.75\ sec$$

$$T_I = \frac{750\ mL}{500\ mL/sec} = 1.5\ sec$$

Flow

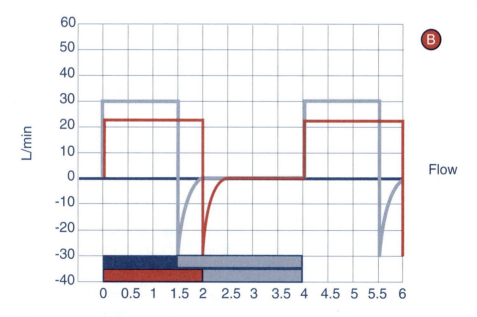

Flow

Figure 1-2A and 1-2B. Effect of changing inspiratory flow rate on inspiratory time and expiratory time.

EFFECT OF CHANGES IN RESISTANCE AND COMPLIANCE

Figures 1-3 and 1-4 demonstrate the effects of changes in airways resistance and decreased respiratory system compliance on the pressure/time scalar.

Pressures plotted on the pressure/time scalar are calculated from the known parameters of R_{AW}, C_{RS}, the inspiratory flow rate, and the delivered tidal volume. During an inspiration and expiration, the gas flow encounters resistance in the airways. The molecular frictional activity results in development of pressure. This pressure is equal to the product of R_{AW} and the gas flow rate. The pressure required to overcome R_{AW} as gas flows through the airways is the transairway pressure (P_{TA}).

$$P_{TA} = \text{flow rate x } R_{AW}$$
$$= 0.5 \text{ L/sec x } 10 \text{ cm } H_2O/L/sec$$
$$= 5 \text{ cm } H_2O$$

Once the gas molecules reach the alveolar region, more pressure is required to deliver a given tidal volume to the lungs against the recoil force of the alveoli. This pressure is known as alveolar pressure (P_A). Since this pressure is obtained from an inspiratory hold or plateau, it is referred to as $P_{PLATEAU}$ or P_{STATIC}. This pressure is calculated from the tidal volume and C_{RS}.

$$P_{PLATEAU} = P_A = \frac{\text{tidal volume}}{C_{RS}}$$

Since the V_T = 750 mL and C_{RS} = 0.05 L/cm H_2O = 50 mL/cm H_2O

$$P_{PLATEAU} = \frac{750 \text{ mL}}{50 \text{ mL/cm } H_2O} = 15 \text{ cm } H_2O$$

Knowing the two pressures, P_{TA} and $P_{PLATEAU}$, the PIP can be obtained.

$$PIP = P_{TA} + P_{PLATEAU}$$
$$= 5 \text{ cm } H_2O + 15 \text{ cm } H_2O$$
$$= 20 \text{ cm } H_2O$$

Figure 1-3 provides a graphical view of increased R_{AW} on the pressure/time scalar. Notice that as the R_{AW} increases the pressure required to overcome airway resistance increases as does the PIP. Initial parameters indicated a P_{TA} = 5 cm H_2O, P_A= 15 cm H_2O and the PIP = 20 cm H_2O. If the airway resistance doubles due to increased secretions, bronchospasm or any other obstruction, the P_{RAW} increases to 10 cm H_2O and the PIP increases to 25 cm H_2O.

Figure 1-4 demonstrates that as the lung compliance decreases the static or plateau pressure increases resulting in increased peak pressure. If the compliance decreases by half (25 mL/cm H_2O), the plateau pressure will increase to 30 cm H_2O and the PIP will increase to 35 cm H_2O.

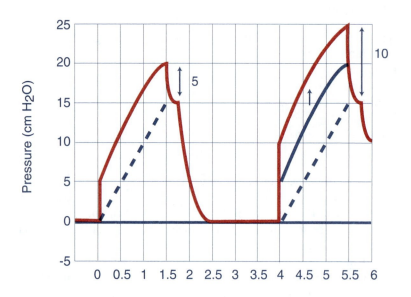

Figure 1-3. The effect of increased airways resistance on the pressure waveform.

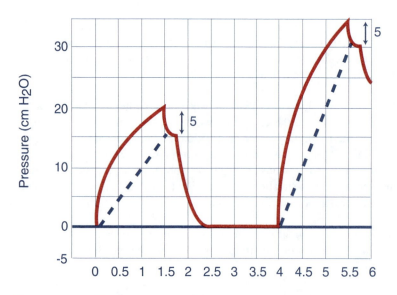

Figure 1-4. The effect of decreased respiratory system compliance on the pressure waveform.

SCALARS

A mechanical breath in a graphical format can be viewed in six stages (Figure 1-5):
  A. Beginning of inspiration
  B. Inspiration
  C. End of inspiration
  D. Beginning of expiration
  E. Expiration
  F. End of expiration

These six stages of a mechanical breath are indicated below:

A. *Beginning of inspiration* depends on the triggering mechanism. In the control mode or in a situation where the ventilator provides backup ventilation, the ventilator initiates mechanical breath on elapse of a predetermined time. This is termed as *time-triggered breath.* In the assist mode or a synchronized intermittent mandatory ventilation (SIMV) mode, the mechanical breath is initiated by the patient's effort. This is termed as *patient-triggered breath.*

B. During *inspiration* the mechanical breath is delivered and the flow, volume, and pressure characteristics of the breath depend on various factors, such as airway resistance, lung compliance, type and magnitude of the flow, and the tidal volume being delivered.

C. The clinicians determine the parameter responsible for *termination of inspiration* referred to as cycling mechanism. These mechanisms include volume cycling, pressure cycling, time cycling, and flow cycling.

D. Generally, during mechanical ventilation, when inspiration ends, the *expiratory phase begins* by opening the exhalation valve. However, in special situations, such as when the inspiratory pause or inflation hold controls are activated, the exhalation valve does not open even though inspiratory gas flow has stopped. The delivered volume is held inside the lungs to obtain static or plateau pressure. Expiration begins in this situation upon opening the exhalation valve. This phenomenon will be demonstrated later in the book.

E. *Exhalation* is passive, and the characteristics of exhalation depend on the airways resistance, the resistance of the artificial airway, and the recoiling force of the lung (compliance).

F. Beginning of the next breath (end of expiration).

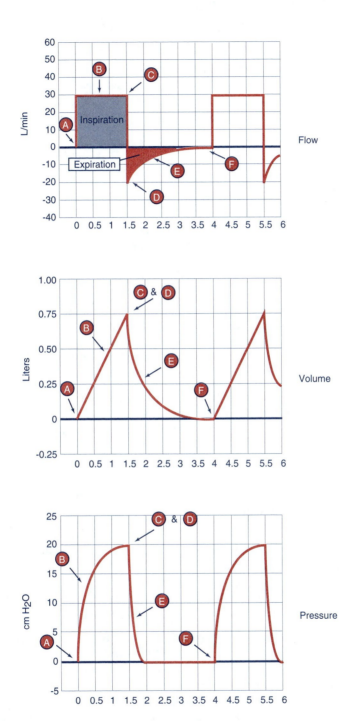

Figure 1-5. Components of the breath cycle.

MODES OF VENTILATION AND CORRESPONDING SCALARS

Figures 1-6 to 1-11 demonstrate the six modes commonly employed in mechanical ventilation. Each set of scalars is shown in two formats: a clean graphic form drawn using the parameters given in the example and an actual waveform generated from a mechanical ventilator graphic module. The reader should compare these two sets of graphics to appreciate the actual and clean versions of the identical waveforms.

CONTROL MODE VENTILATION: Notice the following in Figure 1-6:

a. On each graph the inspiratory time and expiratory times correspond to termination of inspiration and expiration, respectively.

b. *A negative tracing below the baseline is observed during exhalation for the flow/time curve only.* This is because the flow transducer measures inspiratory flow (positive deflection), as well as, expiratory flow (negative flow).

c. The square flow tracing indicates a constant flow pattern.

d. Since the flow is constant, the volume delivery is rectilinear (straight line increase).

e. The initial rise in the pressure to 5 cm H_2O corresponds to the pressure required to overcome airway resistence (P_{TA}). Beyond this point the increase in pressure depends on the lung compliance and the volume delivered up to that point. Near the end of the delivery of tidal volume, the pressure contour has flattened due to delivery of volume in almost filled lungs.

f. At the end of inspiration (1.5 sec) the flow delivery stops, all the tidal volume is delivered, and the peak inspiratory pressure (PIP) has been reached.

Flow vs. Time Scalar: Review Figure 1-6A. At the initiation of mechanical ventilation, the ventilator delivers a constant flow depicted by the square waveform. The flow instantaneously reaches the set level of 30 L/min and continues for 1.5 seconds ($T_I = V_T/flow$). At this time the flow decreases to zero and expiration begins. The transducer reports expiratory flow on the negative side of the scale. This flow reaches its maximum level immediately and tapers up to zero during exhalation. The next inspiration does not begin until the set cycle time ($T_C = 60$ sec/f) of 4 seconds has elapsed and the tracing continues.

Volume vs. Time Scalar: In Figure 1-6B, the monitoring device mathematically performs integration of the flow/time tracing to determine the volume/time tracing. Since the flow rate is constant, the volume is delivered in fixed increments per unit time resulting in a straight line tracing. Volume delivery ends when the set tidal volume of 750 mL is delivered. The exhalation valve opens and volume decays to the baseline. The next volume delivery begins when the cycle time elapses.

Pressure vs. Time Scalar: Look at Figure 1-6C. At the beginning of inspiration, the gas flow experiences the frictional resistance of the airways. Throughout the flow of the gas molecules within the airways molecular bombardment on each other and on the surrounding walls of the airways generates a pressure. The abrupt rise of 5 cm H_2O pressure represents the pressure resulting from the airway resistance (P_{TA} = flow x R_{AW}). After overcoming the frictional resistance, the gas now flows into the alveoli and encounters elastic resistance. Since the inspiratory phase does not terminate until the set tidal volume is delivered, the respiratory compliance promotes a gradual increase in pressure strictly dependent on the volume delivered and the lung compliance ($P_{PLATEAU} = V_T/C_{RS}$). In this case, the plateau pressure of 15 cm H_2O and the P_{TA} of 5 cm H_2O account for the peak inspiratory pressure of 20 cm H_2O. At the end of inspiration (1.5 sec), the pressure decreases to the baseline (zero pressure). The next tracing appears after 4 seconds (T_C).

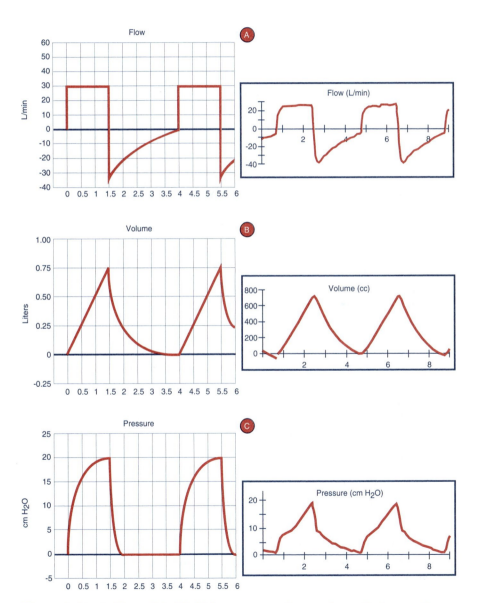

Figure 1-6A, 1-6B, and 1-6C. Volume-targeted control ventilation mode.

ASSIST MODE VENTILATION: Note parameter changes in Figure 1-7. The inspiratory flow was increased to 60 L/min and the ventilator was switched to deliver assisted breaths at 12 breaths/min. However, the patient triggered a rate of 20 breaths/min. Notice that these parameter adjustments also changed other calculated parameters.

$$T_C \text{ decreased to } \quad \frac{60 \text{ sec/min}}{20 \text{ cycles/min}} \quad = \quad 3 \text{ sec}$$

T_I decreased to 0.75 seconds as a result of increased flow rate from 30 L/min to 60 L/min

$$T_I = \quad \frac{750 \text{ mL}}{1000 \text{ mL/sec}} \quad = \quad 0.75 \text{ sec}$$

P_{TA} also increased due to increased flow rate

$$P_{TA} \quad = \text{ flow rate x } R_{AW}$$
$$= 1 \text{ L/sec} \quad x \quad \frac{10 \text{ cm } H_2O}{L/sec}$$
$$= 10 \text{ cm } H_2O$$

And the PIP increases proportionately,

$$PIP = P_{TA} + PA \quad\quad = 10 + 15 \text{ cm } H_2O$$
$$= 25 \text{ cm } H_2O$$

Notice the following:

a. With increased flow, the inspiratory time shortened and allowed the patient to increase the respiratory rate to 20/min. The flow instantaneously reaches to 60 L/min and stays constant for 0.75 sec.

b. A small negative deflection on the pressure/time graph indicates patient triggering characteristic of all assisted breaths.

c. The initial rise of 10 cm H_2O pressure is due to the pressure required to overcome airways resistance. Consequently, the PIP reaches 25 cm H_2O.

Flow vs. Time Scalar: Observe Figure 1-7A. Similar to the control ventilation, the ventilator delivers a constant flow throughout the inspiratory phase as shown by the square wave tracing. Since the flow rate was increased to 60 L/min, flow is maintained at 60 L/min for the duration of the inspiratory time (0.75 seconds). Concurrently, the set tidal volume is delivered and the flow drops to zero and expiration begins. As exhalation proceeds, the flow gradually returns to the baseline. The next inspiration begins after 3 seconds.

Volume vs. Time Scalar: Similar to the volume/time tracing in the controlled mode, volume delivery (Figure 1-7B) is a straight line increase. The delivery of volume is terminated when the set tidal volume of 750 mL is delivered. The exhalation begins and volume decays to the baseline. The next volume delivery begins when the cycle time elapses.

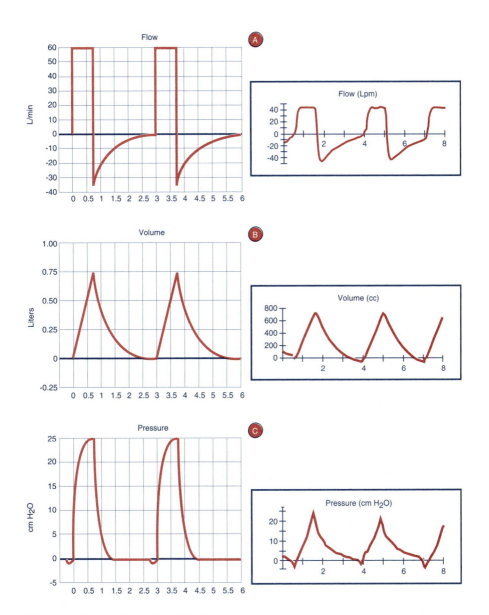

Figure 1-7A, 1-7B, and 1-7C. Volume-targeted assist control ventilation.

Pressure vs. Time Scalar: Note Figure 1-7C. Compared to the pressure/time graph in the controlled mode, certain differences are obvious. A small negative deflection indicates that the breath was initiated by the patient (patient triggering), thus it is called an assisted breath. The first 10 cm H_2O pressure is attributed to the pressure due to the airways resistance (P_{TA} = flow x R_{AW}). Since lung compliance did not change, the pressure required to deliver the tidal volume into the lungs is the same (15 H_2O). As a result, the total peak inspiratory pressure reaches 25 H_2O in 0.75 seconds (inspiratory time). At this time the inspiration ends since the tidal volume is delivered (volume cycling). The exhalation valve opens and the pressure quickly decreases to the baseline.

SYNCHRONIZED INTERMITTENT MANDATORY VENTILATION (SIMV): Note parameter changes in Figure 1-8. On the assisted ventilation at a rate of 20 breaths/min, the patient was hyperventilating. It was decided to place the patient on an SIMV mode with a rate of 12 breaths /minute. This change resulted in an increase in the total rate to 36 breaths/minute indicating that between two mechanical breaths the patient was taking two spontaneous breaths of 150 mL tidal volume.

Notice the following:
a. Between two mechanical breaths, the inspiratory flow tracing on spontaneous breaths is on the positive side of the graph, and during expiratory phase, the flow is registered below the baseline.
b. Spontaneous volume reaches 150 mL.
c. Unlike flow and volume, the inspiratory pressure is traced on the negative side of the baseline and exhalation shows a positive side tracing.
d. The stages in each breath occur at the same points in time in the three scalars.

Flow vs. Time Scalar: Observe that two spontaneous breaths occur in between two mechanical breaths in Figure 1-8A. The mechanical breath has the same characteristics as in the assisted ventilation (Figure 1-7). For the spontaneous cycles, inspiratory flow is shown as a positive deflection and the expiratory flow as a negative contour. Since the SIMV rate is set at 12 /min, the mechanical cycle time is set at 5 seconds. Every 5 seconds, the ventilator delivers a mechanical or mandatory breath.

Volume vs. Time Scalar: The volume delivered during spontaneous breath is only 150 mL where the volume curve reaches the peak (Figure 1-8B). Again, the characteristics of the mechanical breaths are identical to those in the assisted ventilation (Figure 1-7).

Pressure vs. Time Scalar: Notice that the spontaneous breaths are represented by a negative deflection during inspiration and a positive deflection during exhalation (Figure 1-8C). Also, the mechanical breaths are patient triggered as shown by a small negative deflection before the mechanical breath is initiated.

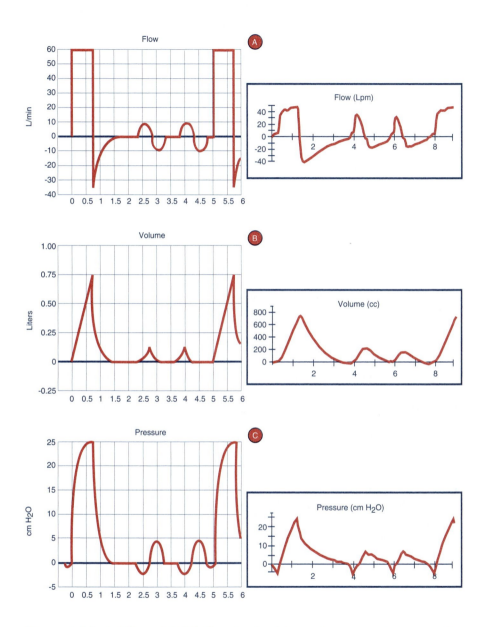

Figure 1-8A, 1-8B, and 1-8C. Synchonized intermittent mandatory ventilation (SIMV) waveforms.

SIMV WITH PRESSURE SUPPORT VENTILATION (PSV): Note parameter changes in Figure 1-9. Since the spontaneous tidal volume was very small, a 10 cm H_2O pressure support was initiated. This manipulation increased the spontaneous tidal volume from 150 mL to 350 mL allowing the patient to decrease respiratory rate from 36/min to 24/min indicating that the patient was interposing one spontaneous breath in between two mechanical breaths.

Notice the following:
a. On the flow/time scalar, the pressure supported breath delivered a decreasing flow and terminated inspiration when the flow reached a certain level (flow cycling).
b. The volume delivery shows that during the spontaneous component of breathing a tidal volume of 350 mL is delivered.
c. Pressure supported breaths are delivered to maintain set pressure (10 cm H_2O in this case) throughout the inspiratory phase. The pressure decays during expiratory phase to the baseline. Also, observe that all breaths are patient triggered confirmed by the small negative deflection to the beginning of inspiration on the pressure/time scalar.

Flow vs. Time Scalar: Notice the pressure supported breath is interposed between two mechanical breaths (Figure 1-9A). The most striking characteristic of the pressure supported breath is its flow delivery. During inspiratory phase the flow tapers from its peak level. A pressure supported breath, generally, terminates inspiration when the inspiratory flow decreases to a system specific flow (usually 25% of the peak flow). Thus a pressure supported breath can be termed as a flow cycled breath.

Volume vs. Time Scalar: As a result of a pressure supported breath the spontaneous volume increased from 150 mL to 350 mL and the spontaneous ventilatory rate decreased (Figure 1-9B). The patient is now initiating only one breath between two mechanical cycles.

Pressure vs. Time Scalar: Observe that the pressure is maintained at 10 cm H_2O throughout the inspiratory phase (Figure 1-9C). Also notice that the spontaneous as well as the mechanical breaths are patient triggered as revealed by the negative deflections on the pressure/time waveform.

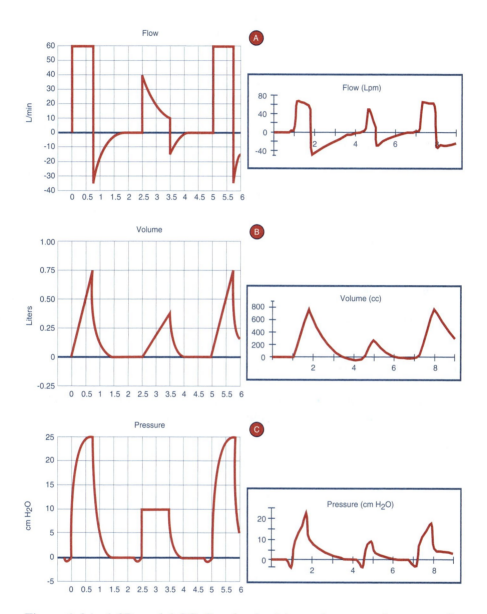

Figure 1-9A, 1-9B, and 1-9C. Synchonized intermittent mandatory ventilation (SIMV) with pressure support ventilation (PSV) waveforms.

SIMV WITH PSV AND CONTINUOUS POSITIVE AIRWAY PRESSURE (CPAP):

Note parameter changes in Figure 1-10. Blood gas analysis indicated that the patient's ventilation was adequate; however, the oxygenation status was not acceptable. The patient showed a PaO_2 of 43 mm Hg on an F_IO_2 of 0.9. It was decided to initiate continuous positive airway pressure (CPAP) to improve oxygenation. Baseline pressures greater than zero are referred to as CPAP in spontaneous breathing, whereas elevated baseline pressures are termed positive end expiratory pressure (PEEP) when mechanical breaths are present. It is becoming common to use the term CPAP for both situtations. CPAP level was gradually increased and titrated with pulse oximetry (SpO_2). At a CPAP level of 15 cm H_2O, the SpO_2 increased to 90%.

Notice the following:
a. Initiation of CPAP elevates the baseline on the pressure/time graph from zero to 15 cm H_2O resulting in the elevation of the peak pressure (PIP) from 25 cm H_2O to 40 cm H_2O.
b. At end of exhalation, the airway pressure decreases to the new baseline of 15 cm H_2O.
c. On flow/time and volume/time tracing, the baseline remains at the same level before instituting CPAP.

Flow vs. Time: Addition of CPAP (Figure 1-10A) does not change the flow pattern from the previous settings (Figure 1-9A).

Volume vs. Time: The volume/time curve (Figure 1-10B) remains unchanged.

Pressure vs. Time: Observe the baseline is elevated from zero to 15 cm H_2O (Figure 1-10C). This resulted in the increase of the PIP from 25 cm H_2O to 40 cm H_2O.

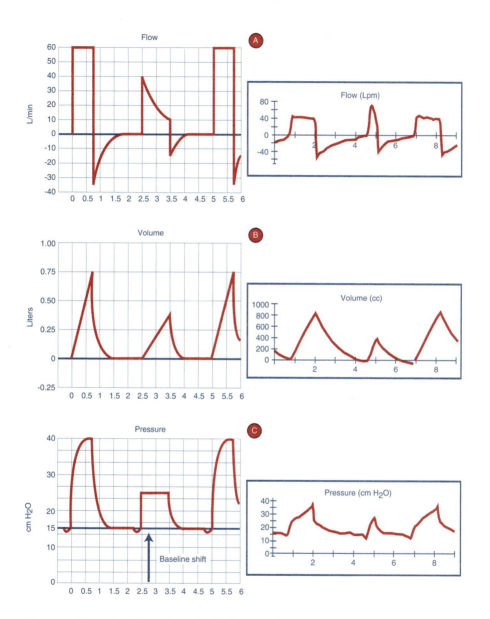

Figure 1-10A, 1-10B, and 1-10C. SIMV with PSV and CPAP.

PRESSURE CONTROL VENTILATION (PCV): Note parameter changes in Figure 1-11. The patient continued to deteriorate. The PIP gradually increased to 55 H_2O. It was decided to switch the patient from volume ventilation to pressure ventilation mode. The patient was sedated, and the ventilator was adjusted to deliver pressure controlled ventilation (PCV) at a level of 30 cm H_2O and at a respiratory rate of 15 breaths/min. The inspiratory time was set to 1.5 seconds and a backup rate at 12/min.

Notice the following:
a. The ventilator terminates inspiration when a preset time has elapsed (1.5 seconds in this case).
b. On the flow/time scalar, the flow decreases to zero before the inspiration ends. The pressure stays at the set pressure throughout the inspiratory time.

Flow vs. Time: Since the pressure control mode is time cycled (Figure 1-11A) mode, the inspiratory flow continues to taper down throughout inspiratory phase and may reach zero flow at or before the inspiratory time (1.5 seconds) elapses.

Volume vs. Time: The delivered volume depends on the lung characteristics (Figure 1-11B). The volume delivery is terminated at the end of inspiratory phase.

Pressure vs. Time: Observe the baseline returns to zero since the PEEP was eliminated (Figure 1-11C). The pressure is maintained at 30 cm H_2O during the inspiratory phase (1.5 seconds).

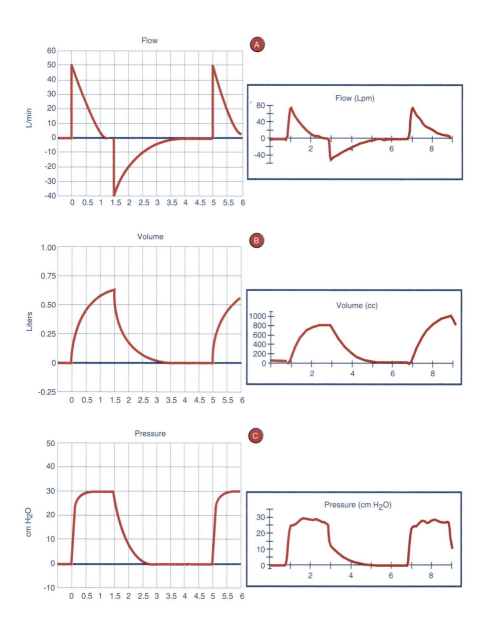

Figure 1-11A, 1-11B, and 1-11C. Pressure control ventilation (PCV).

CHAPTER 2
PRESSURE-VOLUME AND FLOW-VOLUME LOOPS

TOTAL LUNG COMPLIANCE

Pressure-volume (P-V) and flow-volume (F-V) loops are typically studied after becoming familiar with pressure, flow, and volume scalars. As with the scalars, information can be obtained from both numeric values and the shape of the waveforms. A loop is actually an inspiratory and expiratory curve connected together. It is common for clinicians to initially have difficulty with the fact that loops do not express units of time. The progression of a breath can be followed from beginning to end but without any reference to how much time has passed.

It is helpful to have in mind normal patterns, values, and conventions when evaluating P-V and F-V loops. The scale of the axes must be set so that the loops are displayed appropriately for analysis. For example, the P-V loop allows for quickly determining at a glance if a patient's dynamic compliance is abnormal by looking at the slope or pitch of the loop. A loop with normal compliance is conventionally displayed with a slope that is roughly at a 45 degree angle to horizontal. A normal dynamic compliance for a ventilator patient ranges 50-80 mL/cm H_2O (Tobin) so the axes should be set so that a compliance value in the middle of that range (65 mL/cm H_2O) would be at about a 45 degree angle. In some instances, it is helpful to scale the axes without regard for convention so that the screen displays as much of the loop as possible to better see details. Afterward, return the axes scale to a conventional setting so that others can easily monitor patient's graphics even from a distance as they move about a unit or ward. P-V loops in this chapter do not necessarily conform to the 45 degree convention for normal compliance in order to magnify details and display a larger complete graphic.

Most readers may be familiar with F-V loops from pulmonary function studies, but it is important to note that there is no convention for how the inspiratory and expiratory portions of the F-V loops are oriented with respect to horizontal axis. Traditionally, a pulmonary function report displays F-V loops with the inspiratory curve below the horizontal axis and the expiratory curve above the axis. Ventilator graphics displays may show this orientation or the reverse, depending on the brand of equipment. One common source of confusion associated with loop evaluation results from changing more than one ventilator or patient variable at a time. It is helpful to make incremental changes when using ventilatory waveforms to guide fine-tuning of the ventilator to the patient. For example, when trying to assess if a bronchodilator drug had a beneficial effect by comparing changes in the loops before and after treatment, changing the mode of ventilation between measurements may obscure or counterfeit improvements from the drug.

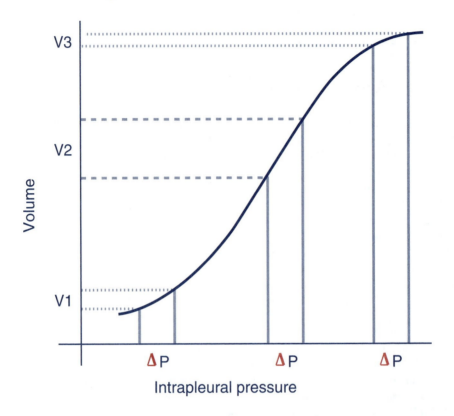

Figure 2-1. Volume as a function of position on the total lung compliance curve.

Compliance is the term commonly used in pulmonary physiology to describe the change in lung volume in relation to the change in intrapleural pressure. There are several specific variations of the term compliance used to discuss ventilatory conditions. The compliance curve produced by slowly inflating a patient's lungs with positive pressure might look similar to the one in Figure 2-1. The largest volume change for a given pressure is obtained at the steepest portion of the curve, the middle. The baseline for tidal breathing is normally positioned in this same region allowing for spontaneous ventilation at the most efficient portion of the curve where the least pressure change is needed. When a pulmonary disorder such as atelectasis or air-trapping significantly increases or decreases, respectively, the baseline for tidal breathing, ventilatory efficiency decreases. This results in decreased dynamic and static respiratory system compliances and distortion of the P-V loop in particular.

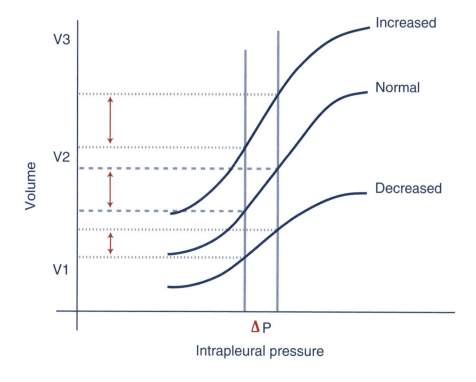

Figure 2-2. Shifts in the lung compliance curve from pulmonary disorders yield different tidal volumes.

Not only are pulmonary disorders able to shift the tidal breathing origin to some abnormally high or low point on the total lung compliance curve, but they can change the shape of the entire curve. Imagine inflating a patient's lungs very slowly so that airways resistance would be almost nonexistent while recording the inspiratory pressure-volume curve. The same pressure change applied to the middle portions of such curves with different slopes would produce different volumes (Figure 2-2).

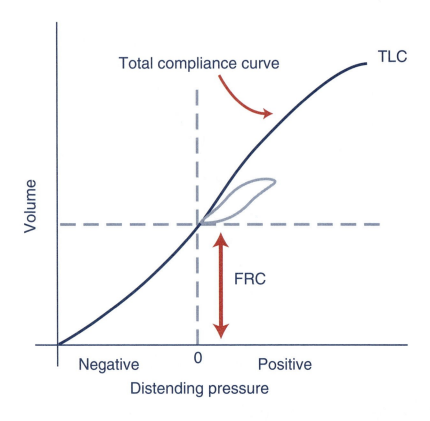

Figure 2-3. The tidal breath in relation to the total lung compliance curve.
(TLC = total lung capacity; FRC = functional residual capacity.)

A positive pressure tidal breath placed on the total compliance curve might look like
the gray loop in Figure 2-3. Functional residual capacity (FRC) is an important term
to understand when discussing relationships in ventilation and respiratory mechanics.
The point of zero airway pressure indicates the balance between the lungs' tendency
to recoil and the chest wall's tendency to expand outward. The volume of gas in the
lungs at this balancing point is the FRC.

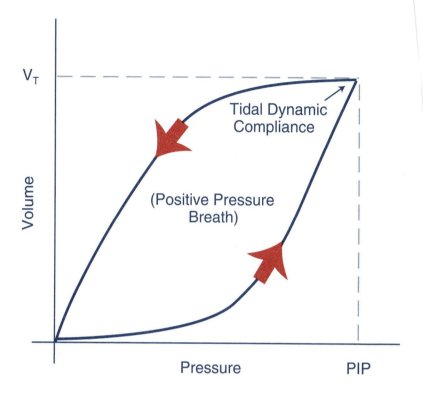

Figure 2-4. Components and labels of a positive pressure breath P-V loop.

Intubated patients are artificially ventilated by positive pressure breaths. When pressure (horizontal axis) and volume (vertical axis) changes are plotted against each other, a loop such as the one in Figure 2-4 is generated. Conceptual renderings of P-V loops are often elliptical or "football shaped" but such a symmetric pattern is not seen in reality. The breath begins in the lower left corner of the graph following the counterclockwise path indicated by the red arrows, finally ending at the lower left corner. The upper right corner of the loop marks the end of inspiration and the beginning of expiration. This point of maximal pressure and volume represents the dynamic compliance (change in volume divided by change in pressure) of the respiratory system for that breath. Note that the loop begins at zero pressure, indicating there is no positive pressure applied to the baseline (PEEP).

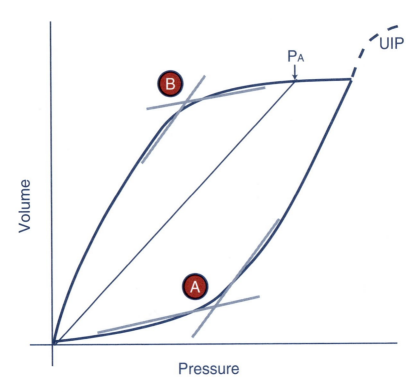

Figure 2-5. Inspiratory and expiratory inflection points of a positive pressure breath. (PA = alveolar pressure).

Changes in respiratory compliance can be detected in the P-V loop by noting changes in the slope of the curve. The point of change in the slope of a line is called the *inflection point*. The loop in Figure 2-5 has two inflection points, one during the inspiratory phase A and one during the expiratory phase B. Point A is referred to as the lower inflection point (LIP) of the inspiratory curve. There can also be an upper inflection point (UIP) during inspiration as indicated by the dashed line if the tidal volume were increased. Point B is the UIP of the expiratory curve (also termed point of maximum curvature [PMC]). A LIP is sometimes seen on expiratory P-V curves. If the inflection point is difficult to determine, it often helps to draw lines along the portions of the inspiratory and expiratory curves that are nearly straight as in Figure 2-5. The point of intersection for the two drawn lines estimates the inflection point. On a static P-V loop, these inflection points are thought to represent a sudden change in alveolar recruitment during inspiration and a derecruitment of alveoli during expiration. Figure 2-5 shows a dynamic P-V loop which includes the effect of resistance to flow. The volume increase lags behind the pressure increase causing a gap between the inspiratory and expiratory curves of the P-V loop. This makes the inflection points obtained from a dynamic P-V loop unreliable for setting PEEP or the upper pressure

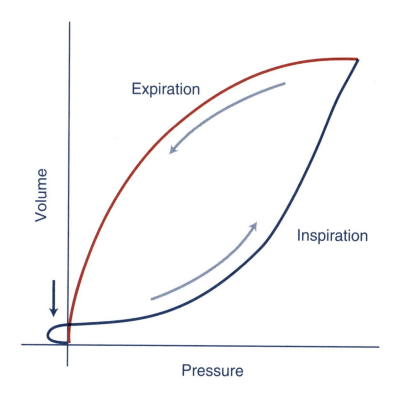

Figure 2-6. Assisted positive pressure ventilator breath.

limit. A more detailed discussion of measuring inflection points and using them to set ventilator controls is given in Chapter Five.

A positive pressure ventilator breath produces a P-V loop similar to the examples in Figures 2-4 and 2-6. Figure 2-4 would represent what is termed a *control breath,* meaning it is triggered solely by the timing mechanism of the ventilator without any regard to whatever spontaneous efforts the patient may have. Figure 2-6 represents a ventilator breath that is triggered by a spontaneous patient respiratory effort. There are many variations of positive pressure breaths, but they will be dealt with in Chapter Three. As previously described, inspiration (represented by the blue line segment) starts at the intersection of the axes in the lower left corner of the graph. The small bulge into the negative side of the pressure axis (see blue arrow) represents the patient's effort to begin inspiration. Spontaneous efforts trace a loop in the clockwise direction. At the point the ventilator senses the patient's effort and starts a machine breath, the line shifts rightward into the positive side of the pressure axis and loops counter clockwise. Expiration starts at point of highest volume and pressure and is represented by the red line segment. Except for the initial patient effort, both inspiratory and expiratory phases of the ventilator breath occur on the positive pressure side of the pressure axis.

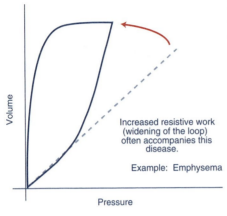

Increased resistive work
(widening of the loop)
often accompanies this
disease.

Example: Emphysema

Figure 2-7. Increased respiratory system compliance.

Recall that the convention for displaying normal dynamic compliance is to have the point of end inspiration displayed so that a line traced to the beginning point of inspiration would be approximately 45 degrees to the horizontal axis (represented by the dotted line in Figure 2-7). An increase in respiratory system compliance causes a shift to the left of the 45 degree line (e.g., less pressure needed to deliver volume).

Patients with emphysema typically have both wide P-V loops and increased compliance with a left shift (Figure 2-7). The widening of the loop is caused by airway resistance which is described later in this chapter. Changes in compliance are not necessarily accompanied by changes in resistance. Increases in compliance often are gradual except in circumstances such as the administration of surfactant therapy.

A decrease in compliance causes a rightward shift in the loop as indicated in Figure 2-8 (more pressure needed to deliver the volume). Variations of this pattern are typically seen in the later stages of acute respiratory distress syndrome (ARDS). Decreases in compliance can occur gradually as in the progression of a pulmonary disease or suddenly such as when large airways become plugged by mucous or by the endotracheal tube advancing into the right mainstem bronchus.

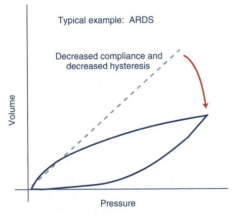

Typical example: ARDS

Decreased compliance and
decreased hysteresis

Figure 2-8. Decreased respiratory system compliance.

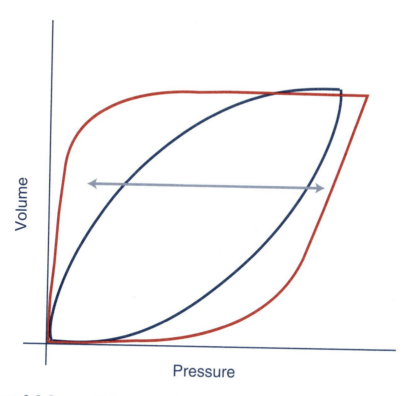

Figure 2-9. Increased airways resistance produces exaggerated P-V loop hysteresis.

Changes in airways resistance cause the area of the P-V loop and its horizontal distance to increase (Figure 2-9). These changes result from hysteresis, a lag in the volume change in relation to the rate of pressure change due to increased airways resistance. Notice that the widened red loop has a greater peak pressure and a slightly lower peak volume than the black loop. The ventilator must apply more pressure to move less volume which indicates a decrease in ventilatory efficiency. The slight rightward shift indicates the resistance is creating a decreased compliance effect. The normal airways resistance range for an intubated patient (up to 5 cm H_2O/L/sec) is slightly higher than for a nonintubated patient (Broseghini). It is difficult for even experienced clinicians to identify increased airways resistance simply by looking at a P-V loop unless the hysteresis is profound or two loops are superimposed for comparison. F-V loops are more commonly used for bronchodilator benefit testing on ventilator patients. However, F-V loops obtained during volume-targeted ventilation do not show inspiratory-only increases in airways resistance well so it is a good habit to review both F-V and P-V loops for changes in airways resistance.

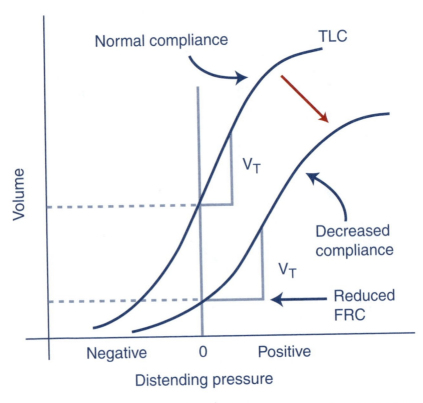

Figure 2-10. Pressure-volume relationship determines work-of-breathing.

The compliance curves in Figure 2-10 are similar to those in Figures 2-1 and 2-2 but show the zero pressure reference point. The importance of FRC to ventilatory efficiency becomes clear when volumes generated for a given pressure change at different points on the total lung compliance curve are compared. The same volume is moved on the normal and low compliance curves but the pressure required to do so is nearly doubled on the curve with decreased compliance. The amount of pressure required to move a particular volume is related to what is termed the *work* done during each breath. The work done during a breath on the rightmost curve is greater due to both the decreased compliance (slope of the curve) and the decreased FRC (position of the zero pressure point on the curve). The work-of-breathing (WOB) can be measured several ways but discussion will only involve the method involving ventilatory graphics also termed *mechanical WOB*.

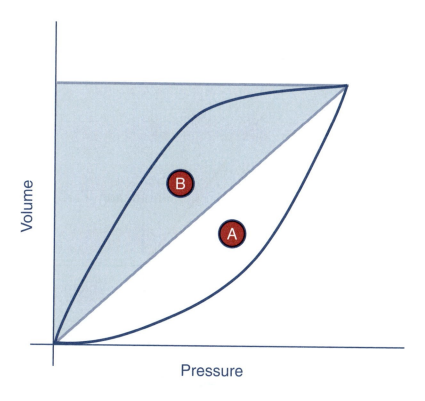

Figure 2-11. The WOB components for a positive pressure breath. (A = Resistive work, B = Elastic work.)

The WOB can be done by the patient, the ventilator, or can be shared by both. The WOB components for a positive pressure ventilator breath are labeled in Figure 2-11. The unshaded portion of the P-V loop marked A represents the WOB due to over-coming airways resistance. The shaded area labeled B represents the WOB required to stretch the elastic lung tissue during inspiration. Together, A and B represent the total mechanical work done during the breath. The WOB is typically expressed as an integral, where WOB equals the area under the changing pressure curve as volume moves from zero to its peak at end inspiration. This may be more clear if you turn the P-V loop 90 degrees to the left so that volume is on the x-axis. The greater the area comprised by A and B, the greater the WOB. Most ventilator graphic displays show only the mechanical work measured at the airway opening (the endotracheal tube connector). This method is reasonably accurate only if the patient is not contributing any ventilatory efforts (essentially paralyzed). Patient contributions to WOB during mechanical breaths can be indirectly measured by plotting esophageal pressures.

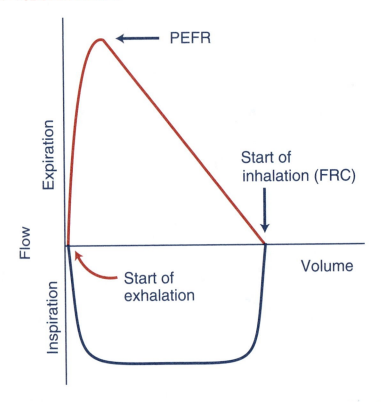

Figure 2-12. Components and labels of a normal positive pressure breath F-V loop.

The F-V loop recorded during mechanical ventilation looks similar to the F-V loop reported in PFT studies, but the two differ in that the mechanical breaths do not represent maximal spontaneous efforts as do the PFT breaths. In Figure 2-12, the vertical axis represents flow rate (liters per second) and the horizontal axis represents volume (usually in liters for adults). The inspiratory portion of the F-V loop (blue) is below the horizontal axis and the expiratory portion (red) is above it. Recall that this orientation may be reversed depending on the brand of equipment. Normally, the transition from inspiration to expiration and back again occurs where the loop crosses the horizontal axis when the flow rate is momentarily zero. The shape of the inspiratory curve will reflect the flow pattern set on the ventilator, which is a constant flow rate or square wave in this case. The highest point above the x-axis represents the peak or maximal expiratory flow rate (PEFR) during a passive exhalation. The shape of this passive expiratory curve will be influenced by anything that may cause airway obstruction.

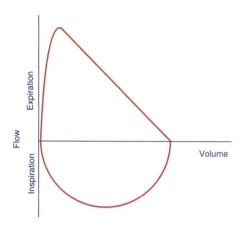

Figure 2-13. Conceptual sinusoidal flow pattern for a positive pressure ventilator breath.

The rendering in Figure 2-13 represents a perfect sinusoidal (sine) pattern that looks similar in shape to those seen in PFT studies. Note that the orientation of the inspiratory and expiratory portions of the loop in Figure 2-14 are opposite of Figure 2-13. The shape can be altered by patient variations, ventilator settings, circuit conditions, and the way in which the breath is generated by the ventilator. Although the peak flow rates are different for the two breaths in Figure 2-14, the shapes are similar. Exhalation is passive, but because this particular ventilator did not deliver the same volume at both flow rate settings, the expiratory flow pattern is slightly altered.

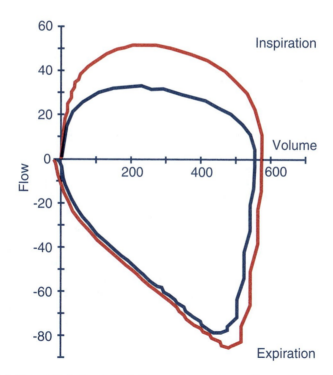

Figure 2-14. Recorded sinusoidal flow pattern at two flow rate settings.

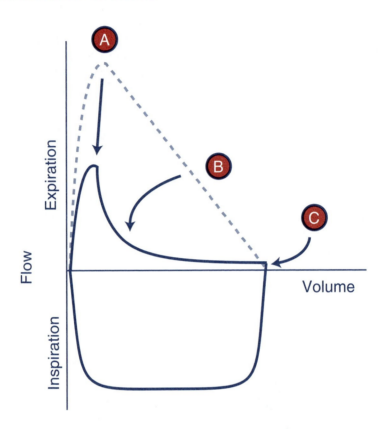

Figure 2-15. Signs of airwary obstruction in the F-V loop.

Airways obstruction can cause several changes in the F-V loop depending on the location and severity. The light blue dashed line in Figure 2-15 represents the normal expiratory flow pattern for the example patient, and the arrows indicate possible deviations from this normal pattern due to obstruction. Most types of significant airways obstruction will reduce the peak expiratory flow rate (arrow A in Figure 2-15). Medium and small airways obstruction also tend to cause the descending segment of the expiratory curve to take on a curvilinear shape (arrow B in Figure 2-15) which is often termed *scooping* in the clinical setting. Air-trapping may occur if expiratory time is insufficient or the smaller airways collapse prematurely due to abnormal anatomic changes. Air-trapping is identified in Figure 2-15 arrow C, the expiratory portion of the loop not returning to baseline (zero flow rate) before the start of the next breath.

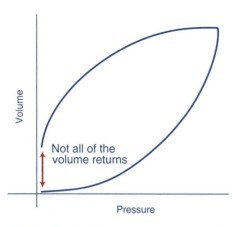

Figure 2-16. Volume loss present in the P-V loop.

Volume loss (e.g., leak) during a breath can be detected in both loop and scalar formats. Volume loss due to some type of leak appears on a waveform as an expiratory volume smaller than the inspiratory volume. The volume lost to leaks that occur downstream from the flow transducer used to generate the loop graphics (on the patient side of the transducer) will appear as part of the inspiratory volume. The lost volume is not returned through the flow transducer so the loop does not close. The gap indicated by the red arrow in Figure 2-16 indicates a partial loss of volume during expiration. Likewise the gap identified by the arrow in Figure 2-17 indicates a volume loss. Possible sources of such leaks include endotracheal tube cuff leaks, bronchopleural fistula, and air leaks through chest tubes. An inspiratory volume that is less than the set volume but has an equivalent expiratory volume would not be due to such a leak. Equally diminished inspiratory and expiratory volumes could be produced by a leak in the ventilator circuit between the flow transducer and the ventilator (e.g., when flow is measured at the proximal airway).

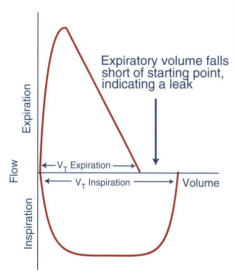

Figure 2-17. Volume loss present in the F-V loop.

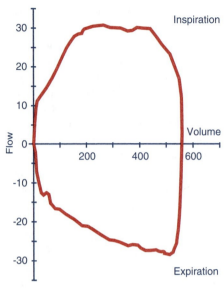

Figure 2-18. Spontaneous breath F-V loop.

Loop waveforms of spontaneous breaths differ in a few ways from positive pressure ventilator breaths. F-V loops are similar except for the inspiratory portion of the loop. The inspiratory curve of a spontaneous breath is rounded, much like a ventilator breath set to the sine wave pattern (Figure 2-14). The principal difference is lower peak flow rate typically observed with quiet spontaneous breathing (Figure 2-18). Expiration is passive so the shape is consistently a descending ramp-like pattern for both spontaneous and ventilator breaths.

The differences between spontaneous and ventilator breath P-V loops are more easily seen. Spontaneous breaths are generated as negative pressure is created in the chest. This causes a leftward bulge of the P-V loop into the negative side of the pressure axis (Figure 2-19). The loop is traced in a clockwise fashion. Exhalation occurs on the positive side of the pressure axis, mirroring the change to positive pressure in the chest and airways during expiration.

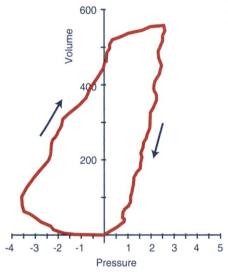

Figure 2-19. Spontaneous breath P-V loop.

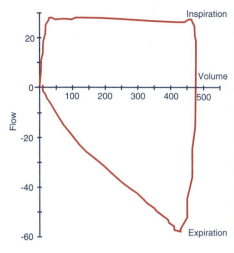

Figure 2-20. F-V loop from a square wave flow pattern positive pressure ventilator breath.

A ventilator breath with a constant flow pattern, also called a *square wave pattern* is displayed in Figure 2-20. The flow rate remains the same throughout most of inspiration. This in turn produces a fairly constant volume delivery. Although this pattern may not be used as often as a descending flow pattern, it is helpful for detecting abnormalities in the P-V loop precisely because flow and volume delivery are constant. Note in Figure 2-21 that the P-V loop has not been scaled to display the slope of a normal dynamic compliance line at roughly a 45 degree angle to the horizontal axis. Recall that a normal dynamic compliance for a ventilator breath ranges from 50-80 mL/cm H_2O. The volume change of 475 mL divided by the pressure change of 13 cm H_2O dynamic yields a dynamic compliance of 37 mL/cm H_2O. The slope of this loop would actually fall below the 45 degree convention. Note the absence of any negative pressure deflection in the P-V loop, thus indicating this is probably a control mode breath.

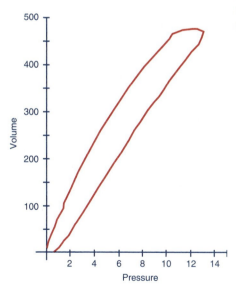

Figure 2-21. P-V loop from a square wave flow pattern positive pressure ventilator breath.

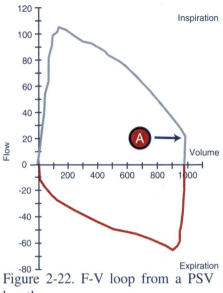

Figure 2-22. F-V loop from a PSV breath.

The PSV breath shown in Figure 2-22 is another type of positive pressure breath. The F-V loop appears at first glance to be two opposing expiratory curves joined together. The inspiratory phase is shown in light blue and the expiratory in red. A PSV breath has a characteristic that can be mistaken for an abnormal clinical condition previously described as air-trapping (Figure 2-15). Note the abrupt change in the slope of the inspiratory curve indicated by point A on the inspiratory curve. This sudden drop toward the horizontal axis at the *end of inspiration* is due to the ventilator cycling from inspiration to expiration at a preselected flow target. Auto-PEEP is identified as a flow above zero at the *end of exhalation*, and the beginning of the next inspiration. Therefore, when inspiratory and expiratory flow patterns look similar, it is especially important to orient yourself as to how inspiration and expiration are displayed on the F-V loop graph.

The P-V loop in Figure 2-23 shows the same PSV breath and color-coding as in Figure 2-22. Note that the inspiratory and expiratory lines cross each other at about +2 cm H_2O instead of at zero on the volume axis (as in Figure 2-6). This crossing of the curves after inspiring 100 mL is due to the patient making a vigorous attempt to inspire during the PSV breath. Therefore the inspiratory curve is not smooth.

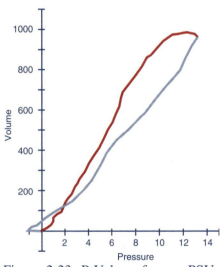

Figure 2-23. P-V loop from a PSV breath.

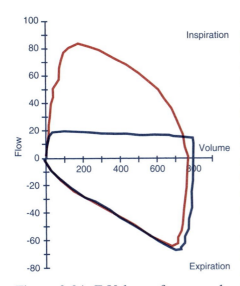

Figure 2-24. F-V loops from a volume-targeted breath (blue) and pressure-targeted breath (red).

A comparison of volume- and pressure-targeted ventilator breaths is shown in Figures 2-24 and 2-25. In both figures, the volume-targeted breath is blue and the pressure-targeted breath is red. The volume-targeted breath has a constant flow pattern which makes it easy to distinguish the inspiratory and expiratory segments of the F-V loop. The pressure-targeted F-V loop is similar to the PSV loop except that it does not have the sudden drop in flow to the horizontal axis at the end of the inspiratory period.

The set pressure for the pressure-targeted breath is similar to the peak pressure observed with the volume-targeted breath (Figure 2-25). Notice that the horizontal diameter and hysteresis are much greater for the pressure-targeted breath. This is not surprising since the flow rate is much higher for this mode throughout inspiration. Also, pressure is relatively constant at about 38-40 cm H_2O. Keep in mind that resistance and compliance for the respiratory system remain the same for both breath types in this example.

It would be inaccurate to attribute the increased hysteresis seen in the pressure-targeted breath as increased airways resistance. That is why it would be inappropriate to change from volume to pressure-targeted ventilation mode or vice-versa between a pre- and post-bronchodilator comparison or while assessing the effect of adjusting other ventilator control variables to fine-tune ventilation.

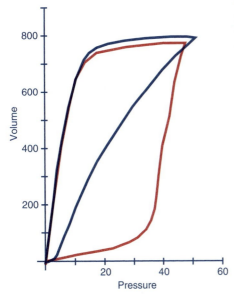

Figure 2-25. P-V loops from a volume-targeted breath (blue) and pressure-targeted breath (red).

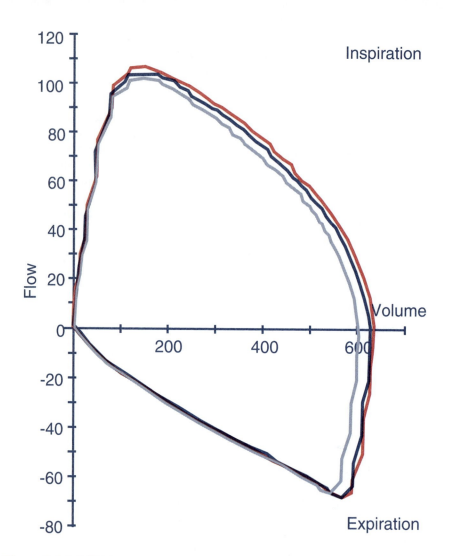

Figure 2-26. PCV breaths with long, short, and no inspiratory pauses.

The F-V loop in Figure 2-26 is enlarged primarily to show the difference in volume between three pressure-targeted breaths with varying inspiratory pauses. The term *inspiratory pause* is somewhat confusing in this case because although the pressure is held constant creating a plateau, volume is allowed to change. The light blue loop represents no inspiratory pause, the blue loop has short pause, and the red loop has the longest pause. In patients that have a wide range of time constants, such as with ARDS, pneumonia, etc., a pressure plateau during a PCV breath can allow for additional volume delivery without increasing pressure. Inspiratory plateaus are also thought to improve distribution of ventilation.

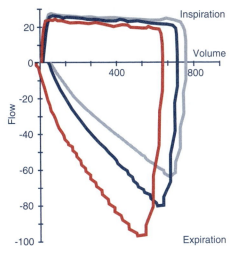

Figure 2-27. The effect of compliance changes on positive pressure breath F-V loops.

Changes in respiratory compliance are best seen in P-V loops, but there are predictable changes that occur in F-V loops as well. A constant flow mode is used in Figure 2-27 to best isolate the effect of changing compliance. Red represents the lowest compliance, blue is a moderate compliance, and light blue is the highest compliance. The tidal volumes increase as compliance increases. Inspiratory peak flows remain similar, but the expiratory peak flow rates decrease as compliance increases. This pattern is related to the concept of elastic WOB described in Figure 2-11. Work is done during inspiration to stretch the elastic tissue in the lung and thorax. The stored force is released during expiration. An increase in compliance is associated with a decrease in the elastic recoil of the lungs. The less elastic recoil present, the less stored energy to be released during exhalation. That is why the peak expiratory flow rates are less as compliance increases.

The P-V graph in Figure 2-28 shows three different respiratory compliances with the same airways resistance value. The light blue loop represents increased compliance, the blue loop represents normal compliance, and the red loop represents decreased compliance. Decreasing compliance is sometimes referred to as a "right-shift" in the P-V loop. Although increased hysteresis can accompany a decrease in compliance they are not linked, as seen in this figure.

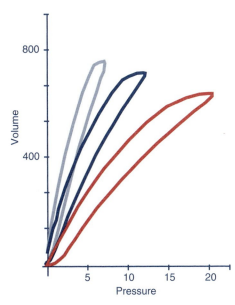

Figure 2-28. The effect of compliance changes on positive pressure breath P-V loops.

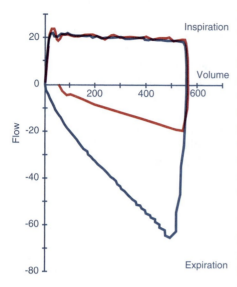

Figure 2-29. F-V loop with normal inspiratory and increased expiratory airways resistance.

Increased airways resistance can occur during inspiration, expiration, or both. The F-V loop in Figure 2-29 contrasts two constant flow breaths, one with normal airways resistance (blue) and the other with increased expiratory airways resistance (red). Notice the decreased peak expiratory flow rate. No scooping is observed, which is consistent with obstruction in the large airways. The shortened return of the red loop indicates a small leak.

The F-V loop for the same breath in Figure 2-30 dramatically shows the effect of increased expiratory resistance. Note that the inspiratory curves are essentially the same, only the expiratory curves differ. Causes of increased resistance during expiration-only include diseases that cause early small airways collapse such as emphysema, bronchomalacia, and the patient biting the endotracheal tube during the expiratory phase.

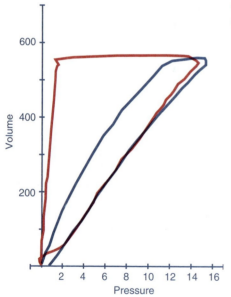

Figure 2-30. P-V loop with normal inspiratory and increased expiratory airways resistance.

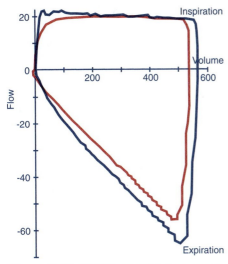

Figure 2-31. F-V loop with increased inspiratory and normal expiratory airways resistance.

The normal loop is in blue and the loop with increased inspiratory resistance is red. The effect of increased inspiratory resistance on the F-V loop in Figure 2-31 is minimal. That is because the driving force of the ventilator is sufficient to overcome the increased resistance. Slightly less volume was delivered so the peak expiratory flow rate was correspondingly less.

The P-V loop in Figure 2-32 impressively shows the increase in inspiratory resistance. The expiratory curves are similar except the volume of the normal curve is slightly greater as observed in the F-V loop. The tidal volume is affected more by inspiratory resistance than expiratory resistance. In ventilator patients, there are few causes of increased resistance during inspiration-only because of the airway-splinting effect of positive pressure ventilation and the endotracheal tube. Examples include the patient biting the endotracheal during inspiration or the rare occurrence of a pedunculated mass (growth attached by a stalk) intermittently blocking an airway, producing a ball-valve effect.

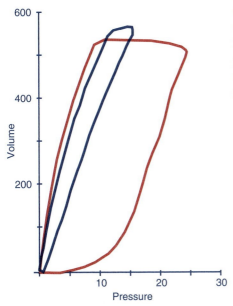

Figure 2-32. P-V loop with increased inspiratory and normal expiratory airways resistance.

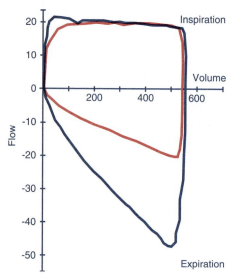

Figure 2-33. F-V loop with both increased inspiratory and expiratory airways resistance.

The two constant flow loops in Figure 2-33 show the combined effects of those in Figures 2-29 and 2-31. The red loop is a result of increases in resistance throughout the entire ventilator breath. Other than a slight rounding of the square inspiratory flow pattern, the only changes from the normal blue loop occur in the expiratory portion.

It is clear that the red P-V loop in Figure 2-34 that corresponds to the red F-V loop in Figure 2-33 reveals more deviations from the normal. Though the increased hysteresis is obvious, without the normal curve present it would be difficult to determine whether it was due to increased resistance during inspiration, expiration, or both. Also, the greater the resistance, the more that volume is decreased from the set value.

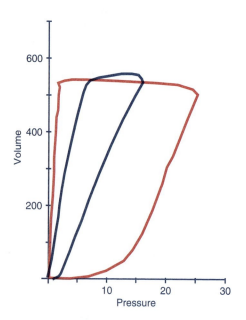

Figure 2-34. P-V loop with both increased inspiratory and expiratory airways resistance.

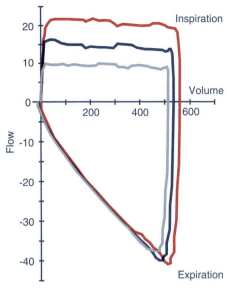

Figure 2-35. F-V loops for volume-targeted positive pressure breaths at three different peak flow rates.

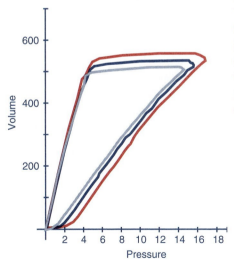

Figure 2-36. P-V loops for volume-targeted positive pressure breaths at three different peak flow rates.

Adjusting peak flow rate in volume-targeted ventilation can produce a variety of changes in ventilator waveforms. It is clear that the flow rate is changing from 20 to 15 to 10 L/min (red, blue, and light blue, respectively). In this particular ventilator, decreasing the peak flow rate resulted in a related decrease in tidal volume. This in turn yielded decreases in expiratory peak flow rate. This fluctuation in the delivered volume in spite of not changing the volume control setting may or may not occur, depending on the brand and model of the ventilator in use.

Flow rate impacts how much resistance develops as a breath is delivered. The progression of P-V loops in Figure 2-36 shows how loop hysteresis decreases as flow rate decreases. With all other variables remaining the same, the decrease in hysteresis that accompanies decreases in flow rate therefore indicates a drop in resistance (P-V loop colors correspond to the F-V loop breaths in Figure 2-35). Therefore, when the flow rate is adjusted to optimize ventilation, such as increasing peak flow rate to extend expiratory time for a patient with airways obstruction, the resulting change in the loop graphic should not be interpreted as a change in the patient's airways.

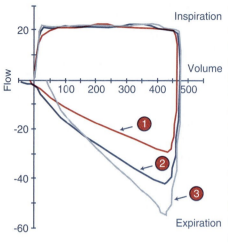

Figure 2-37. F-V loops for volume-targeted breaths with different airways resistances at a compliance of 50 mL/cm H_2O.

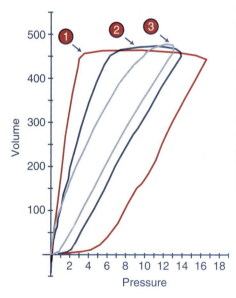

Figure 2-38. P-V loops for volume-targeted breaths with different airways resistances at a compliance of 50 mL/cm H_2O.

The graphic in Figure 2-37 is an example of changing airways resistance with a compliance near the low end of the normal range. If loop 1 represents the condition with the highest resistance, would loop 2 or 3 represent normal? Actually, all three loops represent conditions of abnormally high airways resistance, though loop 3 is only mildly abnormal. Although a single F-V loop can often be used to detect obstruction due to increased airways resistance, it is more useful when loops can be compared over time, or before and after a change or therapy. Notice that as peak expiratory flow decreases, there is no scooping. This suggests that the site of obstruction is in the large airways.

The P-V loops in Figure 2-38 clearly show the increase in hysteresis that accompanies increased airways resistance. Comparing loops 1 and 2 to the condition with the least resistance, loop 3, shows resistance is present on both inspiration and expiration. Waveform monitors that allow loops to be stored in memory for later comparison are very helpful, but small printers can also be used to create printouts for comparisons. Waveform hardcopy from printers is also useful for giving report to colleagues or later creating a case study on an interesting patient.

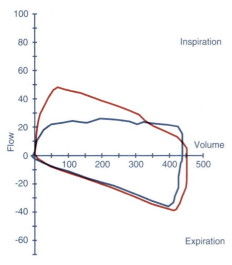

The F-V loops in Figure 2-39 contrast a pressure-targeted (red) and a volume-targeted (blue) breath in the undesirable situation of both increased airways resistance (20 cm H_2O/L/second) and decreased compliance (20 mL/cm H_2O). If the increased resistance is due to bronchospasm and a bronchodilator is administered, the loops in Figure 2-40 result. The resistance decreased to a normal value 2 cm H_2O/L/second) and the compliance remained the same.

Notice that the constant flow inspiratory portion of the volume-targeted breath's F-V loop remains the same but the maximum expiratory flow rate increased. This is expected because the flow rate and pattern are actively controlled in the volume mode whereas expiration is passive and flow rate is influenced by changes in the patient's lungs.

Figure 2-39. F-V loops for pressure and volume-targeted breaths with increased airways resistance and decreased compliance.

The F-V loop for the pressure-targeted breath in Figure 2-39 undergoes changes in both the inspiratory and expiratory segments. Flow rates increase in both phases of the breath and the volume increases slightly, comparing Figures 2-39 and 2-40. This is another way of viewing the effects of changing airway resistance pressure described in Chapter One. (Note the slight leak.)

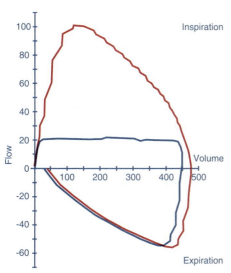

Figure 2-40. F-V loops for pressure and volume-targeted breaths with normal airways resistance and decreased compliance.

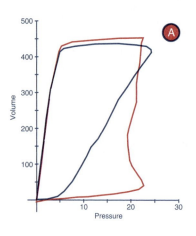

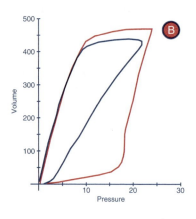

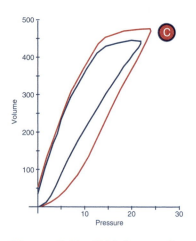

The P-V loops associated with the breaths in Figures 2-39 and 2-40 are depicted in Figure 2-41. The progression from A to C shows the effect of decreasing airways resistance while maintain a low compliance of 20 mL/cm H_2O. More changes occur in the P-V loop when resistance changes so three steps of change are displayed in Figure 2-41. The volume-targeted breaths in A, B, and C (blue) have P-V loops of similar shape except for the hysteresis. The horizontal aspect of the loops appears to shrink proportionately. The pressure-targeted breaths exhibit a less proportional response to changing resistance. Under the highest resistance conditions, the pressure-targeted loop (red) shows an initial bulge that exceeds the pressure at the point of peak volume. As resistance decreases from A to B, the protrusion lessens. From B to C, the primary change is a relatively proportional decrease in the width of the loop. This pattern makes sense when the F-V loops are examined. Recall that the pressure-targeted loop in Figure 2-39 had a much higher flow rate during inspiration, especially at the beginning. Under conditions of normal resistance and compliance the P-V loop of a pressure-targeted breath is very similar to a volume-targeted breath. However, high airways resistance exaggerates the effect of the higher flow pattern for the pressure breath such that the pressure curve begins to follow the pattern of the flow curve.

Figure 2-41. P-V loops alterations during changing resistance.

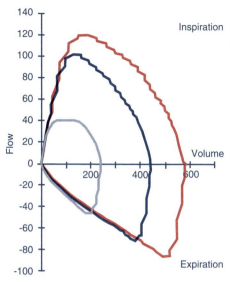

Figure 2-42. The effect of changing pressure levels on F-V loops in PCV mode.

The effect of changing set pressure levels for pressure-targeted breaths produces a predictable pattern as seen in Figure 2-42. As pressure increases, volume increases. Notice the brief plateau in inspiratory flow rate for the loop with the lowest pressure (light blue). A typical ventilator in PCV mode has a high initial flow rate to quickly raise the airway pressure to the set pressure and maintain it for the set inspiratory time. Therefore, peak flow rate is influenced by the conditions of the patient's lungs. Likewise, since only one control variable can be controlled at a time (pressure in this case), volume also changes as flow rate changes.

The P-V loops in Figure 2-43 reveal that resistance and compliance remain fairly constant in this example as peak pressure increases. These P-V loops of pressure-targeted breaths would appear very similar to those of volume-targeted breaths if under the same conditions of low airways resistance. There is no one characteristic shape for a pressure-targeted breath P-V loop. It depends greatly on the conditions in the patient's lungs. The important thing is to understand how the loop shape will change as resistance and compliance change, whether due to changes in anatomy or other ventilator variables.

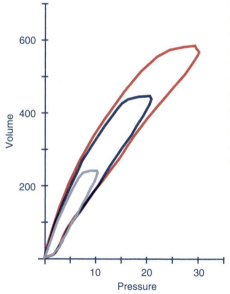

Figure 2-43. The effect of changing pressure levels on P-V loops in PCV mode.

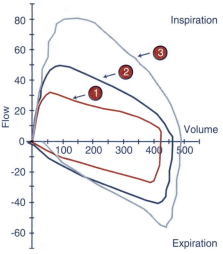

Figure 2-44. The effect of changing airways resistance with normal compliance on F-V loops during PCV.

Final examples of how pressure-targeted F-V and P-V loops can change as a result of different resistance and compliance combinations are given in Figures 2-44 and 2-45. In these examples, compliance is normal for each breath as resistance decreases from loop 1 to loop 3. Notice the sign of air-trapping in loop 1. The F-V loop is constrained to a near rectangular shape as the set pressure is quickly reached due to the increased airways resistance. As resistance decreases, the loops take on more of the typical decelerating ramp pattern.

The P-V loops in Figure 2-45 show a similar pattern as Figure 2-41 but in a superimposed format. In this case, volume increases as resistance decreases. It would be difficult to gauge the degree of resistance if loop 1 or 2 were displayed alone. The goal is to learn how to identify abnormal shapes and compare two or more loops to each other, not to make absolute determinations of the degree of abnormality. Again, the goal is not to memorize shapes but to understand how they are created. This is essential for interpreting the causes of the countless abnormal shapes that are seen in the clinical setting.

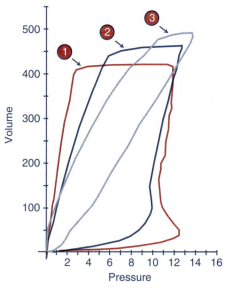

Figure 2-45. The effect of changing airways resistance with normal compliance on P-V loops during PCV.

CHAPTER 3
WAVEFORMS FOR COMMON VENTILATOR MODES

I.   Volume-Targeted Scalars
             Volume-Targeted Control Ventilation
             Volume-Targeted Assist Control Ventilation
             Volume-Targeted SIMV
II.   Pressure-Targeted Scalars
             Pressure-Targeted Control Ventilation
             Pressure-Targeted Assist Control Ventilation
             Pressure-Targeted SIMV
III.   Spontaneous Ventilation Scalars
             Continuous Positive Airway Pressure (CPAP)
             Pressure Support Ventilation (PSV)
             PSV with CPAP
             Setting Rise Time and Flow Cycle Threshold for PSV
             Bi-Level and APRV
IV.   Combination Modes: Volume-Targeted Scalars
             Volume-Targeted SIMV with CPAP
             Volume-Targeted SIMV with PSV
             Volume-Targeted SIMV with PSV and CPAP
V.   Combination Modes: Pressure-Targeted Scalars
             Pressure-Targeted SIMV with CPAP
             Pressure-Targeted SIMV with PSV
             Pressure-Targeted SIMV with PSV and CPAP
VI.   Volume-Targeted Pressure-Volume (P-V) and Flow-Volume (F-V) Loops
             Volume-Targeted Controlled Ventilation with a Constant Flow
             Volume-Targeted Assisted Ventilation with a Constant Flow
             Volume-Targeted SIMV
VII.   Pressure-Targeted P-V and F-V Loops
             Pressure-Targeted Controlled Ventilation
             Pressure-Targeted Assisted Ventilation
             Pressure-Targeted SIMV
VIII.   Spontaneous Ventilation P-V and F-V Loops
             CPAP
             PSV
             PSV with CPAP
IX.   Combination Modes: Volume-Targeted P-V and F-V Loops
             Volume-Targeted SIMV with CPAP
             Volume-Targeted SIMV with PSV
             Volume-Targeted SIMV with PSV and CPAP
X.   Combination Modes: Pressure-Targeted P-V and F-V Loops
             Pressure-Targeted SIMV with CPAP
             Pressure-Targeted SIMV with PSV
             Pressure-Targeted SIMV with PSV and CPAP

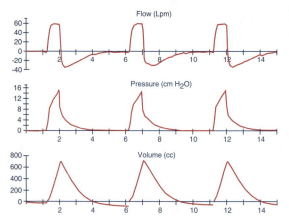

Figure 3-1. Volume-targeted control ventilation.

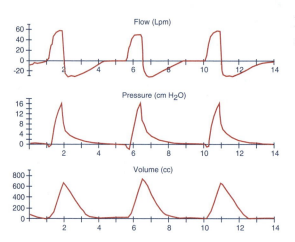

Figure 3-2. Volume-targeted assist control ventilation.

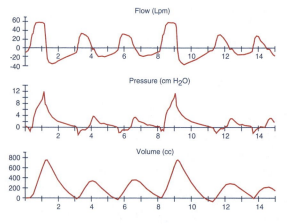

Figure 3-3. Volume-targeted SIMV.

VOLUME-TARGETED VENTILATION SCALARS

VOLUME-TARGETED CONTROL VENTILATION: *Time-triggered, flow-limited, volume-cycled ventilation.* Each breath is a mandatory ventilator breath. Patient triggering does not occur.

Waveform characteristics (Figure 3-1): **Flow/time** scalar indicates a square flow (constant flow). **Pressure/ time** waveform confirms time triggering as each breath is delivered at a fixed time interval (preselected rate on the machine). **Volume/time** scalar displays a linear increase in the volume delivery. The ventilator breath terminates inspiration when the preset tidal volume is delivered (volume cycling). (Note that it is abnormal for the volume waveform to go below the zero baseline. The flow monitor used to calculate volume probably needs to have the calibration reset.)

VOLUME-TARGETED ASSIST CONTROL VENTILATION: *Patient-triggered, flow-limited, and volume-cycled.* Each ventilator breath is triggered by the patient. In the event of apnea, control breaths are delivered at a preset backup rate.

Waveform characteristics (Figure 3-2): **Flow/time** scalar is similar to the control ventilation. **Pressure/time** waveform differentiates a control breath from an assisted breath by the small negative deflection prior to the delivery of the mechanical breath. The assisted breath can be either pressure or flow triggered. *The pressure/time tracing is the only scalar that identifies a patient- (pressure) triggered breath.* **Volume/time** scalar shows a fixed tidal volume being delivered. Regardless of rapid triggering rate by the patient the delivered tidal volume does not change.

VOLUME-TARGETED SIMV: Spontaneous breaths are interposed between mechanical breaths. Preselected mechanical breaths (set by the rate control) are delivered at preset tidal volumes. The patient is allowed to breath spontaneously in between the mechanical breaths.

Waveform characteristics (Figure 3-3): **Flow/time** graphics demonstrate mechanical breaths delivered at a constant flow rate. The spontaneous breaths are indicated by lower flows and nonconstant flow patterns. There are two spontaneous breaths interposed between each mechanical breaths. **Pressure/time** scalar demonstrates two low pressure tracings (spontaneous breaths) between two higher pressures associated with the mechanical breaths. Observe that the mechanical breaths are assisted and synchronized breaths as demonstrated by a small negative deflection before the breath is delivered. The negative pressure of the spontaneous breath reflects inspiration, whereas the positive pressure on the tracing is associated with expiration. **Volume/time** tracing displays smaller volumes delivered during spontaneous component of the SIMV cycle.

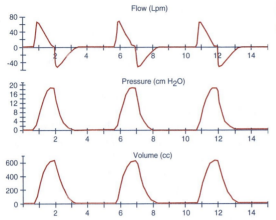

Figure 3-4. Pressure-targeted control ventilation.

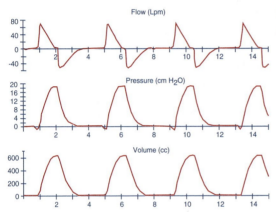

Figure 3-5. Pressure-targeted assist control ventilation.

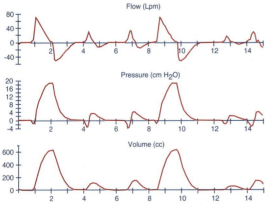

Figure 3-6. Pressure-targeted SIMV.

PRESSURE-TARGETED VENTILATION SCALARS

PRESSURE-TARGETED CONTROL VENTILATION: *Time-triggered, pressure-limited, time-cycled ventilation. (Although pressure cycled is a type of pressure targeted ventilation it is rarely used and therefore not addressed in the remaining text.)* Each breath is a controlled mechanical breath. This mode can be employed for ventilating patients in acute respiratory failure, especially in situations where the lung compliance is decreased.

Waveform characteristics (Figure 3-4): **Flow/time** scalar helps identify a pressure controlled breath. Each breath is delivered at a fixed time interval. The flow descends throughout inspiration. The inspiratory phase terminates when the preset inspiratory time elapses (time cycling). **Pressure/time** scalar shows a sustained pressure (plateau) at the preset pressure level. This combination with the flow pattern can be used to identify a PCV breath. **Volume/time** tracing is similar to the pressure/time curve in that the volume plateau is commonly observed. The volume decline occurs upon opening of the exhalation valve when the preset inspiratory time has elapsed.

PRESSURE-TARGETED ASSIST CONTROL VENTILATION: *Patient-triggered, pressure-limited, time-cycled ventilation.* Each breath is a ventilator breath triggered by the patient (pressure or flow triggered). In the event of apnea, control breaths are delivered at a preset backup rate.

Waveform characteristics (Figure 3-5): **Flow/time** tracing is consistent with that during control pressure ventilation. The flow gradually tapers down to the baseline during the inspiratory time. Occasionally, the flow falls to the baseline before the inspiratory time has elapsed . However, in such a case, the exhalation valve does not open and a zero flow state is observed. **Pressure/time** scalar shows a small negative deflection prior to delivery of a mechanical breath consistent with the triggering effort made by the patient. Each breath in this example is patient triggered. The pressure plateaus until the inspiratory time is over. **Volume/time** tracing is similar to the control breath.

PRESSURE-TARGETED SIMV: All mechanical breaths are delivered as preselected pressure control breaths (assisted) with interposed spontaneous breaths. Each breath is patient triggered breath, unless the patient becomes apneic, at which time the controlled breaths are delivered at the preselected backup rate.

Waveform characteristics (Figure 3-6): **Flow/time** tracing shows the pressure control breaths (assisted) with characteristic descending flow pattern. Notice that exhalation does not begin until the set inspiratory time has elapsed. **Pressure/time** pattern shows a pressure plateau during mechanical breaths. The spontaneous breaths are identified from the inspiratory pressure below the baseline and the expiratory pressure above the baseline. **Volume/time** waveform indicates an increased delivery of volume, a volume plateau, and a decline to the baseline during mechanical breaths. Note the smaller volume for spontaneous breaths.

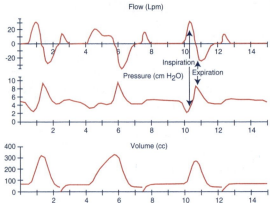

Figure 3-7. CPAP scalars.

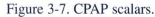

Figure 3-8. PSV scalars.

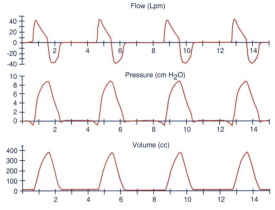

Figure 3-9. PSV with CPAP scalars.

SPONTANEOUS VENTILATION SCALARS

CONTINUOUS POSITIVE AIRWAY PRESSURE (CPAP): A commonly employed mode used to increase functional residual capacity (FRC) in patients demonstrating refractory hypoxemia who are able to maintain adequate spontaneous ventilation. In obstructive sleep apnea, CPAP assists in keeping the upper airways open.
Waveform characteristics (Figure 3-7): **Flow/time** curve simply indicates inspiratory and expiratory spontaneous flows**.** **Pressure/time** is the tracing that identifies the presence of CPAP, which is the spontaneous ventilation baseline maintained at a positive pressure. **Volume/time** shows variable spontaneous volumes.

PRESSURE SUPPORT VENTILATION (PSV): This mode augments a spontaneous breath by applying a preselected pressure to deliver a higher volume at a lower patient effort. Most suitable to overcome the work-of-breathing associated with artificial airways and ventilator circuitry during a spontaneous breath.
Waveform characteristics (Figure 3-8): **Flow/time** waveform is used to recognize a pressure supported breath. The descending flow waveform abruptly drops to baseline at a system-specific terminal flow (more clearly seen in Figure 3-9). **Pressure/time** tracing indicates a patient triggered breath. The pressure rises to the preset level and plateaus until the flow cycling occurs. **Volume/time** shows delivered volume which depends on the pressure support level.

PSV WITH CPAP: A mode used to decrease spontaneous work-of-breathing and support oxygenation. This mode may be used with or without an endotracheal tube. This mode used without an endotracheal tube is termed Noninvasive Positive Pressure Ventilation (NPPV). Common applications include home care use in COPD patients, sleep apnea patients nonresponsive to CPAP therapy, and nocturnal ventilatory assistance to patients with nueromuscular disorders.
Waveform characteristics (Figure 3-9): **Flow/time** tracing is similar to flow/time pressure support-only tracing. CPAP is not detected in this scalar. **Pressure/time** scalar identifies an elevated baseline (CPAP) and pressure support level. **Volume/time** waveform is consistent in this example but can vary depending on patient effort.

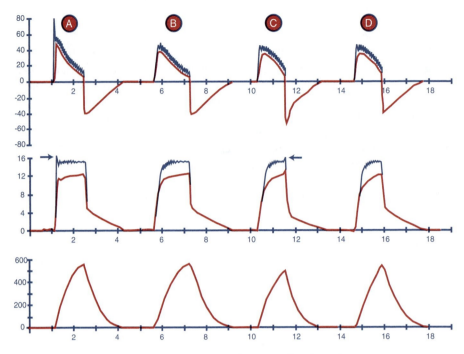

Figure 3-10. The effect of rise time setting on PSV breaths.

Breath A in figure 3-10 shows the effect of increased resistance to flow (i.e., small artificial airway, partially obstructed airway) during a PSV breath. The red tracing was measured at the patient ET-Tube whereas the blue tracing was measured within the (adult) ventilator. The arrow identifies a pressure spike that can occur when resistance is increased or the rise time slope is set too high. Likewise a flow spike can be seen at the beginning of inspiration. In adults these artifacts are usually seen only when measuring at ventilator side of the circuit. In breath B the rise time slope has been decreased to remove the initial spike however as Marcelo Amato has noted, "Since most of this pressure overshoot represents pressure dissipation as frictional work across endotracheal tube, it does not cause elevation of peak alveolar pressure and is probably not associated to any harm." An insufficient rise time slope is of greater concern because it can lead to increased work-of-breathing (WOB) and dyssynchrony with the patient. Increasing rise time slope or the set pressure is often helpful (ventilator flow performance tends to be poor in most ventilators at set pressures < 10 cm H_2O). Breath C shows an end-inspiratory spike (arrow) in the pressure scalar due to active exhalation causing early termination of inspiration. By setting the expiratory trigger at a higher percentage of peak inspiratory flow (increasing the flow cycle threshold) as seen in breath D, the spike is eliminated. This may improve patient-ventilator synchrony and reduce inspiratory muscle effort or it may decrease V_T and worsen blood gases so monitor the patient's response carefully.

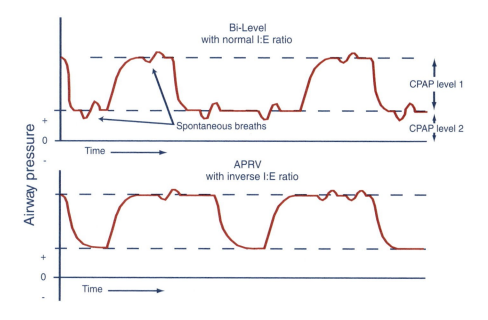

Figure 3-11. Bi-Level and APRV comparison.

Both bi-level and airway pressure release ventilation (APRV) allow two levels of CPAP to be set. Spontaneous breathing can occur at both pressure levels. Ventilation is assisted when the patient is released from the higher CPAP level to the lower CPAP level. Bi-Level ventilation can have a normal or inverse I:E ratio, whereas the APRV implies an inverse I:E ratio. Spontaneous breaths can also be pressure supported in bi-level (or Bi-Level™) ventilation. The goal when setting APRV is to set the lower pressure level time (T_{LOW}) short enough to prevent alveolar collapse. This typically means a T_{LOW} of less than one second and/or evidence of slight auto-PEEP.

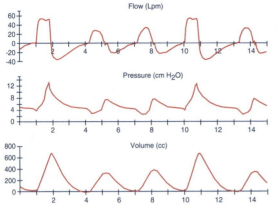

Figure 3-12. Volume-targeted SIMV with CPAP scalars.

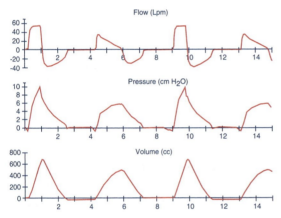

Figure 3-13. Volume-targeted SIMV with PSV scalars.

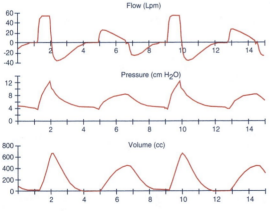

Figure 3-14. Volume-targeted SIMV with CPAP and PSV scalars.

COMBINATION MODES:
VOLUME-TARGETED VENTILATION SCALARS

VOLUME-TARGETED SIMV WITH CPAP: Delivery of SIMV breaths at a higher baseline pressure. Each breath, mechanical or spontaneous, is patient triggered with a positive pressure baseline. Patients in hypoxemic respiratory failure, unresponsive to oxygen therapy, may benefit from SIMV with CPAP.
Waveform characteristics (Figure 3-12): **Flow/time** curves indicate the same pattern as SIMV without CPAP. The mechanical and spontaneous breaths are displayed at a higher baseline pressure. **Volume/time** tracing is similar to a SIMV volume waveform.

VOLUME-TARGETED SIMV WITH PSV: The spontaneous breaths are augmented by an addition of pressure support. All breaths are patient triggered.
Waveform characteristics (Figure 3-13): **Flow/time** graph demonstrates square flow pattern for mechanical breaths. In this case, the flow/time tracing is a way to identify pressure supported breaths. The pressure supported breaths are indicated by the decreasing flow pattern with an elevated set pressure. The spontaneously triggered (patient triggered) pressure supported breaths are flow cycled whereas the mechanical breaths are volume cycled. **Pressure/time** scalar demonstrates two distinct pressure/time waveforms during a SIMV breath and a pressure supported breath. The PSV breath illustrates a more rounded pressure curve as compared with the smooth rising pressure during the inspiratory phase of the SIMV breath. The flow/time scalar can be used to differentiate PSV breaths from constant flow mechanical breaths, but the pressure/time scalar can indicate both PSV and CPAP. **Volume/time** curve indicates the volume differences during the two breaths.

VOLUME-TARGETED SIMV WITH CPAP AND PSV: This mode allows delivery of SIMV and PS breaths at a higher baseline pressure.
Waveform characteristics (Figure 3-14): **Flow/time** tracing is similar to SIMV with PSV scalar. **Pressure/time** waveform identifies presence of CPAP. **Volume/time** scalar is similar to the SIMV and PSV scalar.

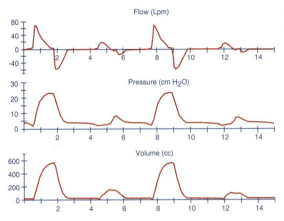

Figure 3-15. Pressure-targeted SIMV with CPAP.

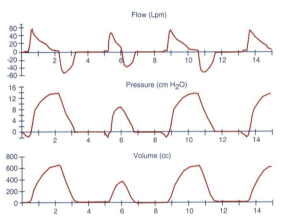

Figure 3-16. Pressure-targeted SIMV with PSV.

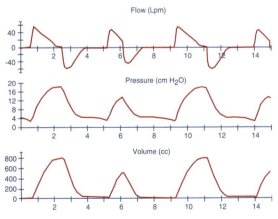

Figure 3-17. Pressure-targeted SIMV with CPAP and PSV.

COMBINATION MODES:
PRESSURE-TARGETED VENTILATION SCALARS

PRESSURE-TARGETED SIMV WITH CPAP: Delivery of SIMV breaths at a higher baseline pressure. Each mechanical breath is an assisted pressure controlled breath (time cycled) interposed by spontaneous breaths. Each breath is patient triggered. The mechanical breaths are delivered at a preselected positive pressure.
Waveform characteristics (Figure 3-15): **Flow/time** scalar indicates the same pattern as SIMV in pressure targeted ventilation. **Pressure/time** tracing indicates CPAP pressure. The pressure tracing does not return to zero. Mechanical and spontaneous breaths are displayed at a higher baseline pressure. **Volume/time** scalar is similar to the volume-targeted SIMV only volume scalar.

PRESSURE-TARGETED SIMV WITH PSV: Spontaneous breaths are augmented by an addition of preselected pressure. All breaths are patient triggered.
Waveform characteristics (Figure 3-16): **Flow/time** graph demonstrates characteristic descending flow pattern for both the pressure control mechanical breaths and pressure support breaths. Observe that in a pressure controlled breath the flow descends steadily until the baseline is reached, followed by a short no-flow state. Whereas in the pressure support breath, the flow descends to a point where inspiration terminates at a specific flow value (flow cycled) and then flow abruptly drops to the baseline. The flow/time tracing along with the pressure/time tracing is the best way to identify pressure controlled and pressure support breaths. **Pressure/time** scalar demonstrates the two distinct pressure/time waveforms: a pressure targeted SIMV breath and a pressure supported breath. **Volume/time** curve simply indicates the volume differences during the two breaths. In fact, if the pressure level is adjusted to match the tidal volume delivered during the SIMV breath (PSV_{MAX}), the volume/time curve would show no significant difference in delivered volumes if patient characteristics remain stable.

PRESSURE-TARGETED SIMV WITH CPAP AND PSV: This mode allows a delivery of SIMV breaths at a higher baseline pressure and pressure support level.
Waveform characteristics (Figure 3-17): **Flow/time** tracing is exactly like the SIMV (pressure targeted) with PSV mode and does not give any clue regarding the CPAP addition. **Pressure/time** waveform clearly identifies the presence of CPAP and the magnitude of CPAP. The presence of PSV is noted on the flow/time scalar whereas the pressure/time scalar indicates PSV and CPAP. **Volume/time** scalar is similiar to the volume/time scalar seen with PC-SIMV with PSV tracing.

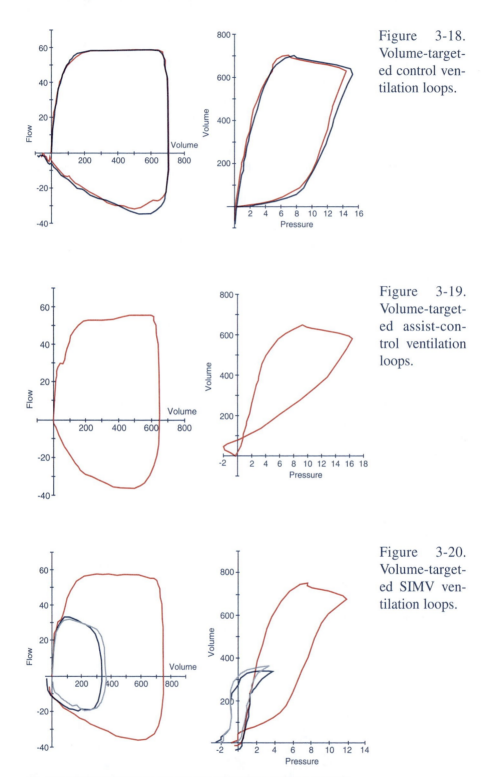

Figure 3-18. Volume-targeted control ventilation loops.

Figure 3-19. Volume-targeted assist-control ventilation loops.

Figure 3-20. Volume-targeted SIMV ventilation loops.

VOLUME-TARGETED VENTILATION
PRESSURE -VOLUME AND FLOW-VOLUME LOOPS

VOLUME-TARGETED CONTROLLED VENTILATION WITH A CONSTANT FLOW: **Flow-Volume (F-V) loop** demonstrates a square wave flow pattern during inspiration (above the volume axis) and exhalation is shown in the bottom part of the loop (Figure 3-18). The flow quickly increases from zero to the preset peak flow rate and remains unchanged until the inspiratory phase is terminated when the preset tidal volume is delivered (volume-cycled ventilation). Upon termination of inspiration the flow decreases at the baseline to the level of peak expiratory flow rate then ends upon return to the baseline (zero flow). **Pressure-Volume (P-V) loop** represents a loop characterized by constant volume delivery. The tracing begins at the zero origin and concludes at the same point.

VOLUME-TARGETED ASSISTED VENTILATION WITH A CONSTANT FLOW: **F-V loop** (Figure 3-19) is similar to the control mode loop. **P-V loop** illustrates patient triggering. The loop begins at zero. When the loop moves to the left of the volume axis this indicates an inspiratory effort made by the patient. When this effort is detected by the ventilator, a mechanical breath is delivered. The loop then moves to the right of the volume axis and returns to zero during exhalation. The spontaneous effort is traced in a clockwise fashion and the mechanical breath is traced counter-clockwise. The negative movement to the right of the volume axis represents patient assist (pressure).

VOLUME-TARGETED SIMV: **F-V loop** shows two types of breaths (Figure 3-20). The smaller, inner loops represents spontaneous breaths with smaller volumes, whereas the larger loop represents a mechanical breath. **P-V loop** tracing includes a smaller P-V loop representing spontaneous breathing (which would be a clockwise tracing on the negative side of the pressure axis). The larger loop illustrates a mechanical breath.

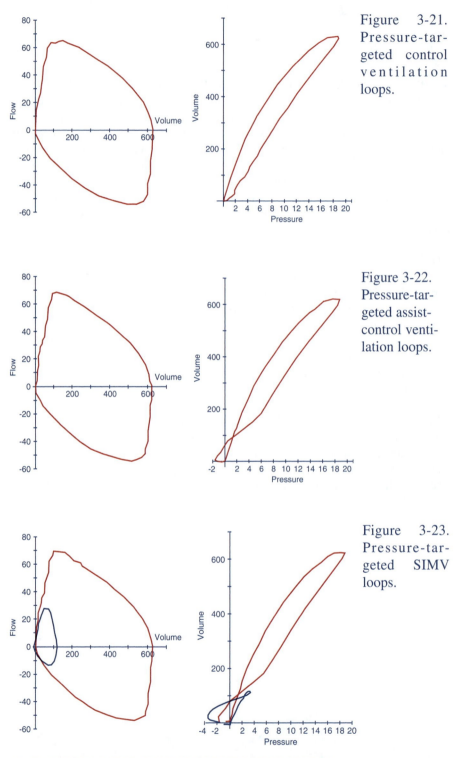

Figure 3-21. Pressure-targeted control ventilation loops.

Figure 3-22. Pressure-targeted assist-control ventilation loops.

Figure 3-23. Pressure-targeted SIMV loops.

PRESSURE-TARGETED VENTILATION
P-V AND F-V LOOPS

PRESSURE-TARGETED CONTROLLED VENTILATION: Pressure control mode delivers a time-triggered, pressure-limited, time-cycled breath (Figure 3-21). The inspiratory flow descends during inspiration to maintain the target pressure until the preset inspiratory time elapses. The expiratory flow is descending. **F-V loop** illustrates a descending inspiratory as well as expiratory flow. **P-V loop** demonstrates a smaller (thinner) hysteresis compared to volume ventilation with constant flow. The descending flow is responsible for the smaller hysteresis of the P-V loop.

PRESSURE-TARGETED ASSISTED VENTILATION: Pressure control ventilation in assist mode delivers a patient-triggered, pressure-limited, time-cycled breath (Figure 3-22). **F-V loop** shows a tracing similar to control ventilation, a descending pattern in both inspiration and expiration. **P-V loop** indicates a negative deflection on the pressure axis consistent with the triggering effort made by the patient.

PRESSURE-TARGETED SIMV: **F-V loop** shows two magnitudes (Figure 3-23). A smaller loop represents a spontaneous breath and a larger loop illustrating a mechanical breath. **P-V loop** also illustrates a smaller spontaneous loop and a larger loop associated with a mechanical breath. The smaller negative pressure deflection represents the patient's triggering the machine breath. The slightly larger blue loop encompassing the smaller red negative pressure deflection represents the spontaneous breath. The largest loop on the positive pressure side represents the machine breath.

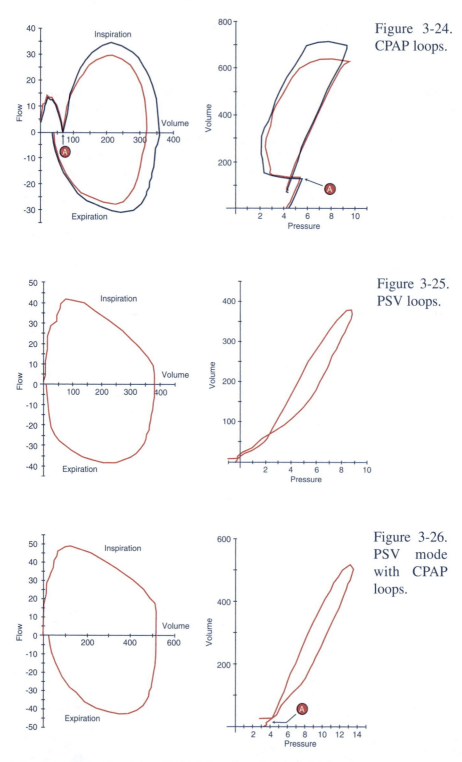

Figure 3-24. CPAP loops.

Figure 3-25. PSV loops.

Figure 3-26. PSV mode with CPAP loops.

CPAP: **F-V loop** shows some deviation from the zero volume point during exhalation due to a leak in the circuit (Figure 3-24). At the beginning of inspiration, the flow rate drops momentarily to zero (item A) before completing inspiration. CPAP is not reflected on the F-V loop. **P-V loop** clearly illustrates that the pressure volume tracing originates at a higher pressure and returns to nearly the same point at the end of the breath. This pressure variance is indicative of CPAP. Item A in the P-V loop corresponds to item A in the F-V loop. Volume increases briefly with a positive increase in pressure, and then pressure decreases for the remainder of inspiration. This type of inspiratory beginning is likely due to excessive response by the flow compensation setting.

PSV: **F-V loop** illustrates a descending inspiratory flow rate until a system specific flow is achieved, then the flow rate rapidly decreases to zero (Figure 3-25). The unusually rounded expiratory portion of the loop continues until the lung volume and flow return to zero. **P-V loop** illustrates patient triggering, then the pressure support breath is delivered with expiration returning to zero baseline. The loop moves in a clockwise pattern during the initial phase (patient triggering) of the pressure support breath and then counterclockwise for the mechanically delivered pressure support breath.

PSV WITH CPAP: **F-V loop** tracing representing PSV and CPAP is similiar to Figure 3-25 which represents the F-V loop for PSV mode (Figure 3-26). **P-V loop** is similar to P-V loop for PSV except the point of origin and the point of termination for this loop is at a higher pressure level indicating CPAP.

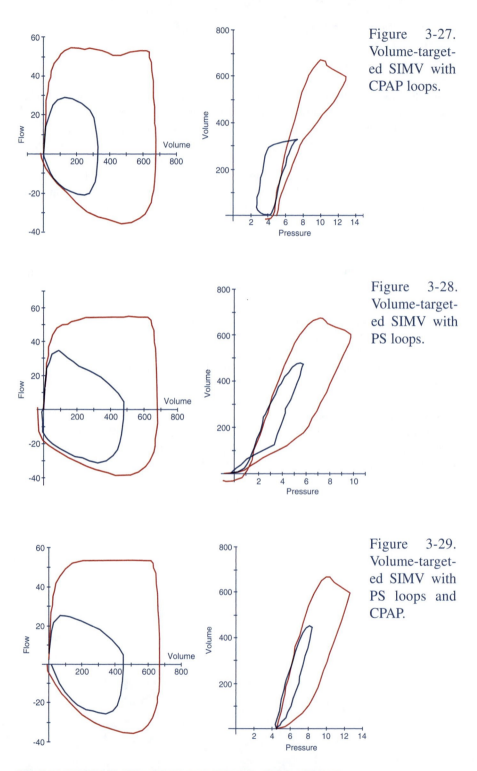

Figure 3-27. Volume-targeted SIMV with CPAP loops.

Figure 3-28. Volume-targeted SIMV with PS loops.

Figure 3-29. Volume-targeted SIMV with PS loops and CPAP.

COMBINATION MODES:
VOLUME-TARGETED VENTILATION P-V AND F-V LOOPS

VOLUME-TARGETED SIMV WITH CPAP: **F-V loop** is similar to Figure 3-20 indicating two distinct loops, one a mechanical breath and the other a spontaneous breath (Figure 3-27). **P-V loop** has a similar appearance as Figure 3-20, except that the zero point is moved to a positive pressure level consistent with CPAP.

VOLUME-TARGETED SIMV WITH PSV: **F-V loop** shows two types of tracings: a PSV tracing (smaller loop) and a mechanical breath (larger loop) (Figure 3-28). The mechanical breath is an assisted breath similar to Figure 3-19. **P-V loop** is essentially a combination of a tracing similar to Figure 3-25 superimposed onto Figure 3-19. The two breaths are separate types, and seeing them together in Figure 3-28 provides practice in distinguishing the two.

VOLUME-TARGETED SIMV WITH PSV AND CPAP: **F-V loop** does not indicate any presence of CPAP (Figure 3-29). It shows a similar pattern as the F-V loop in Figure 3-28. **P-V loop** is similar to Figure 3-28 except CPAP is present.

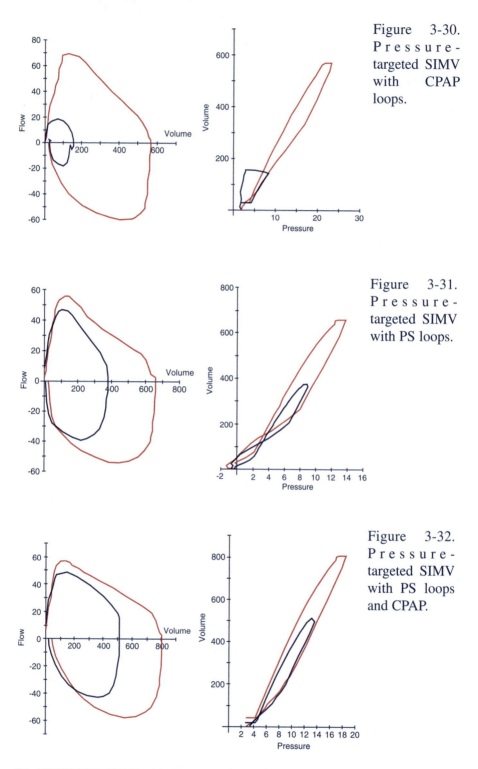

Figure 3-30. Pressure-targeted SIMV with CPAP loops.

Figure 3-31. Pressure-targeted SIMV with PS loops.

Figure 3-32. Pressure-targeted SIMV with PS loops and CPAP.

COMBINATION MODES:
PRESSURE-TARGETED VENTILATION P-V AND F-V LOOPS

PRESSURE-TARGETED SIMV WITH CPAP: The SIMV breath begins at a higher baseline pressure indicating the presence of CPAP (Figure 3-30). **F-V loop** shows distinct loops representing an SIMV breath in pressure control mode similar to Figure 3-22 and a spontaneous breath. **P-V loop** has a similar appearance to the P-V loop in Figure 3-22, except for the higher baseline pressure representing CPAP.

PRESSURE-TARGETED SIMV WITH PSV: Figure 3-31 shows two types of tracings: a PSV tracing and a mechanical breath. The mechanical breath (higher volume and flow tracing) is an assisted breath similar to Figure 3-22. The smaller loop represents a PS breath similar to Figure 3-25. **P-V loop** provides a tracing that would be similar to superimposing Figure 3-22 onto Figure 3-25. The larger loop represents the machine breath and the smaller loop represents the PS breath.

PRESSURE-TARGETED SIMV WITH PSV AND CPAP: **F-V loop** does not indicate any presence of CPAP (Figure 3-32). It shows an identical pattern as the F-V loop in Figure 3-31. **P-V loop** is similar to Figure 3-31 except the zero point is advanced to a higher level illustrating a presence of CPAP.

CHAPTER 4
MONITORING PRESSURE AND VOLUME VENTILATION

INTRODUCTION

Mechanical ventilation has evolved from early volume-targeted ventilators such as the Emerson Post-op and Bennett MA-1 to providing the now common approach of combining volume- and pressure-targeted controls. Traditional volume ventilation has been found not to be the most protective approach for fragile patients such as those with ARDS. Some now advocate starting with pressure-targeted ventilation when possible (Marini) (Houston), but the consensus recommendation is to at least use low tidal volumes (see bibliography).

Volume-targeted ventilation refers to the delivery of a preset volume to the patient. Upon delivery of this volume the ventilator terminates inspiration (volume cycling). On the other hand, pressure-targeted ventilation delivers a preset pressure for a pre-set inspiratory time (pressure cycling is another type of pressure-targeted ventilation but is rarely used). Inspiration is terminated when the set inspiratory time elapses (time cycling). In volume ventilation, patient changes in airway resistance and lung compliance result in corresponding changes in driving pressure required to deliver a preset tidal volume. In pressure ventilation these variations in lung characteristics do not affect the preset pressure, but result in changes in the delivered volume.

Clinical applications of volume- and pressure-targeted ventilation require a thorough understanding of these modes. It is imperative that a clinician in the critical care setting be familiar with both types of ventilation. To protect the lungs from overdistension and the resulting damage from shear forces, the alveolar pressure (estimated by $P_{PLATEAU}$) should be kept below 30 cm H_2O, regardless of the mode of ventilation used (ARDSNetwork).

Pressure varies with volume-targeted ventilation, dependent on the lung characteristics and the caliber of the circuit. Setting the desired tidal volume based on ideal body weight is a common practice; however, current data indicates that higher tidal volumes even in normal range may promote overdistension and may be detrimental to the lungs. This is especially likely for conditions such as in ARDS where the majority of a set tidal volume may be delivered to the small portion of the lungs remaining with a normal compliance. Pressure ventilation is generally indicated for these patients. Volume ventilation has its role in patient populations that do not exhibit low lung compliance. It may be easier to maintain stable blood gas values with volume-targeted ventilation when patient compliance and resistance are frequently (albeit modestly) changing. Generally, short-term, post-operative patients, neuromuscular patients, and drug overdose patients can be better managed by volume ventilation, whereas patients with decreased lung compliance such as ARDS require pressure ventilation to prevent overdistension.

The goal of volume-targeted ventilation is to titrate the $PaCO_2$ to the patient's normal level and support ventilation at a minimal work-of-breathing for the patient. When appropriately set, pressure-targeted ventilation helps protect the lung from overdistension and can be programmed for recruiting maneuvers to reopen areas of collapsed alveoli. The mean airway pressure can be manipulated with less chance of overdistending the lung when using pressure-targeted ventilation. A clinician is expected to be familiar with the type of ventilation the patient is receiving and all monitoring aspects associated with the ventilator-patient interactions. This chapter compares ventilator waveforms during different volume and pressure-targeted ventilation conditions.

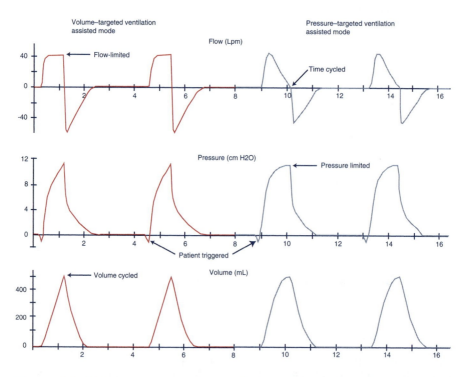

Figure 4-1. Volume vs. pressure ventilation scalars. Volume-targeted and pressure-targeted examples set to deliver similar tidal volumes at similar patient resistance and compliance values.

The examples in Figure 4-1 show flow, pressure, and volume scalars for the same patient using first a volume-targeted mode and then a pressure-targeted mode. Volume ventilation allows the use of a square, descending, or sine wave flow pattern, (some ventilators offer additional patterns). Regardless of the flow pattern, inspiration is terminated when the preset tidal volume is delivered. The graphic shows a square wave or constant flow pattern. During pressure-targeted ventilation, the clinician sets a desired inspiratory pressure and inspiratory time. The inspiration is terminated when the set inspiratory time elapses. Since the pressure gradient between the preset limiting pressure and alveolar pressure decreases as the lung begins to fill, the flow is always descending after the initial peak.

The pressure scalar for the volume-targeted breath has a curvilinear shape dependent on the lung characteristics of resistance and compliance. The peak inspiratory pressure (PIP) varies according to changes in lung characteristics. The consistent peak pressure for the pressure-targeted mode often (but not always) exhibits a square shape for the inspiratory pressure/time curve that indicates the PIP is independent of lung characteristics and will maintain the desired preset pressure.

Comparison of the volume scalar for volume-targeted ventilation vs. pressure-targeted ventilation reveals that the curve is rectilinear in volume-targeted ventilation (due to square flow pattern) whereas it has a curvilinear shape in pressure-targeted ventilation. Recognize that the delivered volume will remain relatively constant in volume-targeted ventilation, but it will vary in pressure-targeted ventilation as lung characteristics change.

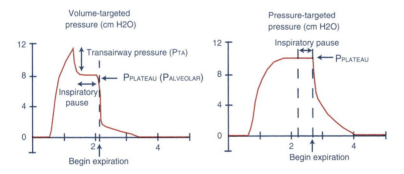

Figure 4-2. Observed inspiratory pause during both types of ventilation (zero flow during end inspiration).

Observe the gradient between PIP and $P_{PLATEAU}$ (transairway pressure) in the pressure scalar of the volume-targeted breath in Figure 4-2 when an inspiratory pause occurs. If during a pressure-targeted breath the inspiratory flow returns to baseline (zero flow) before the end of inspiration, this effectively creates an inspiratory pause. In this case, the alveolar pressure and the airway pressure have equilibrated indicating no transairway pressure gradient and therefore no associated resistance at that moment. The PIP in this circumstance is representative of the end inspiratory alveolar pressure and therefore relates to the respiratory system compliance.

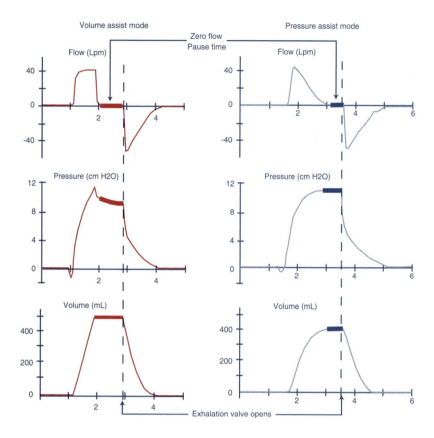

Figure 4-3. A contrast of ventilator scalar changes in volume-targeted vs. pressure-targeted ventilation with an inspiratory pause.

During volume-targeted ventilation, an inspiratory pause causes a rapid decrease of flow to the baseline, and it stays at a zero state until the pause time elapses at which time the exhalation valve opens and exhalation proceeds (Figure 4-3). A zero flow state at the end of inspiration during the pressure-targeted breath is observed which corresponds with an inspiratory pause. The volume scalar shows the volume held in the lungs during the inflation hold for both the volume-targeted and pressure-targeted breaths. It is necessary to view the flow scalar to determine if an inspiratory pause is occurring during pressure-targeted ventilation, i.e., a flow of zero at the end of inspiration.

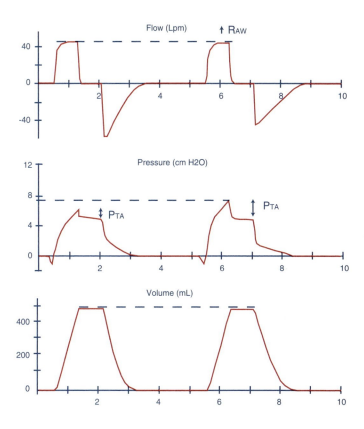

Figure 4-4. Shows the effect of increased airways resistance on volume-targeted breaths.

In Figure 4-4, the second breath shows how the gradient between the PIP and $P_{PLATEAU}$ (transairway pressure) increased as a result of the increased airways resistance. Notice that the delivered tidal volume and peak flow remained constant. An increase in airways resistance during volume-targeted ventilation promotes an increase in the PIP and no change in $P_{PLATEAU}$ (an increased transairway pressure).

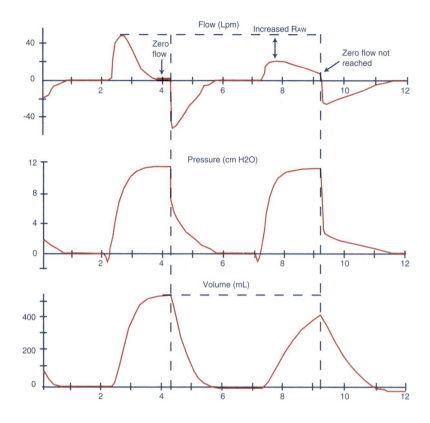

Figure 4-5. The effect of airway resistance on pressure-targeted ventilation.

EFFECTS OF INCREASED AIRWAY RESISTANCE ON VOLUME AND PRESSURE-TARGETED VENTILATION: An increase in airway resistance during pressure-targeted ventilation precipitates several changes: a slower rate of flow deceleration and a decreased peak flow due to resistance and delivery of smaller tidal volume. Notice in the second breath of Figure 4-5, the flow does not return to the baseline in the flow scalar and the volume scalar indicates a decreased tidal volume. A volume plateau is reached with the lower resistance (first breath), but the volume of the second breath (higher resistance) continues to increase throughout inspiration.

In pressure-targeted ventilation, the pressure will always be limited to the set pressure and will not exceed the set pressure irrespective of increase in the airways resistance. Notice that the shapes of the inspiratory pressure curves for the two resistance conditions are similar despite the marked changes in the flow and volume waveforms. The predominant effect of increased airway resistance during pressure ventilation is the concomitant decrease in the delivered tidal volume.

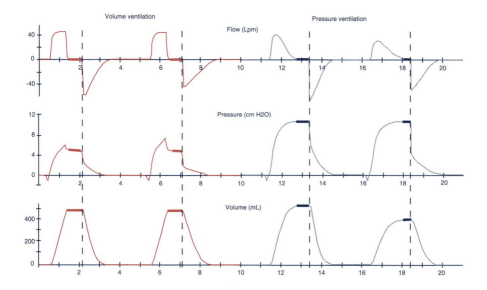

Figure 4-6. Changes due to increased resistance in volume- and pressure-targeted ventilation are contrasted.

In Figure 4-6, the inspiratory flow waveform changes for pressure-targeted but not volume-targeted breaths. The plateau pressure remains unchanged as the transairway pressure increases for the volume-targeted breath, while the pressure-targeted breath is less likely to reach zero flow and the associated inspiratory pause. The volume-targeted breath maintains a constant volume and the pressure-targeted breath yields a smaller volume.

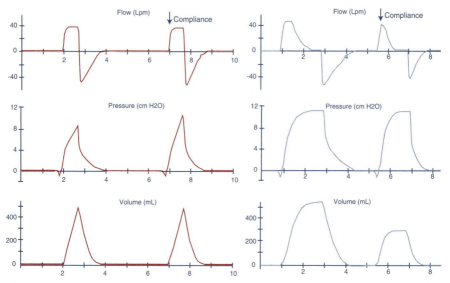

Figure 4-7. The effect of decreased compliance.

EFFECT OF DECREASED COMPLIANCE: In Figure 4-7, observe how the PIP increases in volume-targeted ventilation. The peak expiratory flow is slightly greater and returns to the baseline more quickly due to the increased lung recoil, but the delivered tidal volume is unchanged. If an inspiratory pause were activated, an increased plateau pressure would also be seen. With a pressure-targeted breath, decreased compliance hastens the descent of the inspiratory flow curve to the baseline before the set inspiratory time has elapsed, often creating a no-flow period. This creates the inspiratory pause effect previously described (Figure 4-3). In contrast to the volume-targeted breath, the pressure-targeted example does not show an increased peak expiratory flow. In addition, the tidal volume is reduced as a result of the decreased compliance.

THREE CONDITIONS IN PRESSURE-TARGETED BREATHS: Now notice the three conditions for pressure-targeted breaths in Figure 4-8. All breaths have the same inspiratory time but somewhat different flow tracings. Example A shows the flow scalar with an optimal inspiratory time for the patient conditions. Example B shows the effect of decreasing lung compliance as indicated by the return of inspiratory flow to the baseline before the inspiratory time has elapsed. Example C illustrates increased airways resistance causing slower descent of inspiratory flow resulting in termination of flow before the preset inspiratory time elapses.

It is interesting to note that the flow scalars of two other breath types appear to be similar to example C in Figure 4-8. These are the pressure support breath and a volume-targeted breath with descending ramp flow pattern in Figure 4-9.

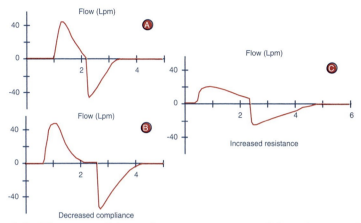

Figure 4-8. Three conditions for pressure-targeted breaths are displayed together.

The three breath types having different cycling variables can have similar flow curves depending on the patient conditions and control settings. It is important to properly set the low volume alarm during pressure-targeted ventilation since it will alert the clinician when the delivered tidal volume decreases due to increased resistance or decreased compliance (similar to high pressure alarm in volume-targeted ventilation).

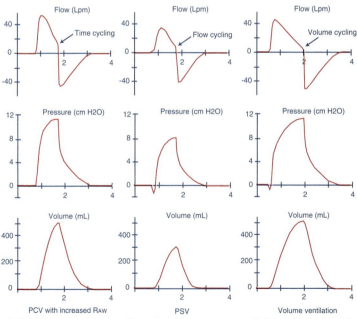

Figure 4-9. Pressure-targeted and volume-targeted breaths with decending ramp flow.

CHAPTER 5
COMMON CLINICAL FINDINGS

I.   Changes in Respiratory System Compliance
          Decreased Compliance and Inflection Points
          Overdistension
          Active Exhalation

II.   Airway Obstruction
          Bronchospasm: Bronchodilator Benefit Assessment
          Air-trapping from Dynamic Hyperinflation
          Air-trapping from Early Small Airway Collapse
          Kinked Endotracheal Tube

III.   Patient-Ventilator Dyssynchrony
          Inadequate Inspiratory Flow Rate
          Inappropriate Trigger Sensitivity
          Patient and Ventilator Rates Out of Synchrony

IV.   Leaks

There are many possible abnormal ventilator waveform variations but the most common findings make a relatively short list. The following specific examples are arranged under the general categories to which they relate.

CHANGES IN RESPIRATORY SYSTEM COMPLIANCE

DECREASED COMPLIANCE AND INFLECTION POINTS

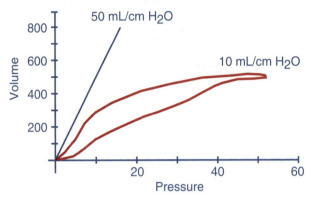

Figure 5-1. The P-V loop of a patient with severely decreased respiratory compliance.

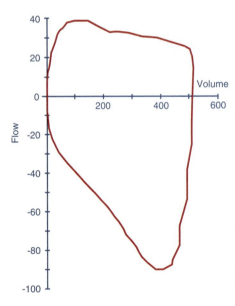

Figure 5-2. The F-V loop of a patient with severely decreased respiratory compliance.

Decreased respiratory compliance is best appreciated in the P-V loop (Figure 5-1). The blue line indicates the slope for the low end of the normal compliance range. The loop has a dynamic compliance of 10 mL/cm H_2O and is shifted downward and to the right of the normal compliance line. The F-V loop corresponding to this patient example is essentially normal except for the relatively high expiratory flow rate for a tidal volume of 500 mL (Figure 5-2). The F-V loop does not provide much information for this particular patient condition, but it is given in this instance for orientation purposes.

The goal of determining best or optimal PEEP for ventilator patients has been pursued by many approaches. It has traditionally sought the best balance between indicators of oxygenation, cardiac function, and respiratory mechanics. The lung protective approach to setting PEEP is to maximize recruitment of alveoli to restore FRC and prevent cyclic derecruitment injury without causing alveolar overdistension. PEEP is used to maintain an open (inflated) lung. As PEEP is increased, the tidal volume must be decreased to prevent excessive alveolar pressures. Many of the publications in the bibliography at the end of this book describe rationales for selecting optimal PEEP. The purpose of this text is to explain how techniques involving waveforms are performed and interpreted, not to argue the efficacy of the techniques.

The pressure-volume curves discussed in Chapter Two are dynamic waveforms. This means they are plotted as gas is flowing during a breath. Static pressure-volume plots can be created by incrementally inflating and deflating the lungs with sufficient pauses between each increment to reach a steady pressure. This is time-consuming and usually requires some form of temporary paralysis making it impractical for most clinical environments. In addition, oxygen consumption during slow inflation maneuvers (lasting more than 30 seconds) introduces significant measurement error. A more clinical-friendly variation of this can be done by inflating the lungs at a constant, very low flow (i.e., less than 10 L/min) corrected for known airway resistance so that the resulting plot is similar to a static plot (even this method may require some sedation). This "quasi-static" curve will often (but not always) reveal inflection points that possibly can be used to guide the setting of PEEP (inflection point identification can sometimes be difficult without computer-assistance). One approach is to set the PEEP level slightly above the lower inspiratory inflection (LIP) point. Some advocate setting PEEP by the expiratory curve inflection point. Still others recommend that inflexion points should not be used and that other measures such as dynamic inspiratory compliance, the linear or "best" compliance (middle portion of the inspiratory curve), or decremental PEEP trials should be used. Such debate is beyond the scope of this text, and no consensus currently exists.

The plots in Figure 5-3 show examples of dynamic, static, and quasi-static pressure-volume curves from the same patient. As previously mentioned, if this approach to setting PEEP is used, the static curve would be preferred but is often not feasible. The quasi-static curve may be a satisfactory substitute and the LIP is estimated by noting the change in compliance as indicated in the figure. The dynamic curve is shown for comparison sake to reveal its inadequacy for determining the LIP.

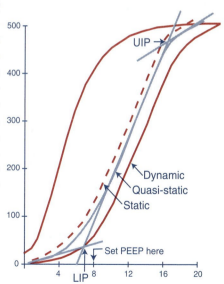

Figure 5-3. P-V loop inflection points.

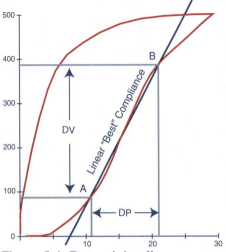

Figure 5-4. Determining linear compliance from a P-V loop.

Figure 5-4 shows a pressure-volume plot identifying the linear compliance of the inspiratory curve. Setting PEEP to produce the highest compliance measured from this linear portion of the inspiratory P-V curve is yet another approach to setting optimal PEEP. The P-V curve can be generated by using a constant pressure increase (i.e., 3 cm H_2O/sec) or a low constant flow. Regardless of what method is used to set optimal PEEP, a lung recruiting maneuver should always be done before and after a PEEP trial (a lower PEEP is needed once the lung is opened). The more common lung recruitment methods to date involve using a CPAP level from 35-50 cm H_2O for about 30-40 seconds. Another variation on using compliance to set ventilator parameters involves using compliance based on the end inspiratory pressure in PCV mode (which is similar to a plateau pressure during an inspiratory pause) to determine optimal PIP and PEEP. First, an attempt is made to recruit as much lung volume as possible starting at a high PEEP level (15-20 cm H_2O) and then increasing PIP (in PCV mode) after a few breaths at each small step until reaching 50 cm H_2O. Once the lung is opened, the PIP is then set at a pressure that will produce a V_T of 5-7 mL/kg ideal body weight (IBW) as the PEEP is changed in small decrements. As the PEEP decreases, compliance increases because some of the overinflated alveoli are relieved. Eventually the compliance plateaus and

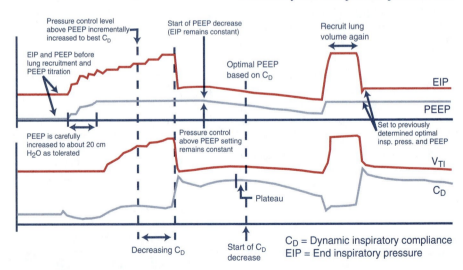

Figure 5-5 Setting optimal PEEP and EIP guided by compliance.

then begins to decrease as alveoli begin to close. The PEEP is set above the point of decreasing compliance. The whole procedure takes about 10-12 minutes. The best inspiratory compliances measured during the incremental PIP and decremental PEEP maneuvers and the associated pressures are used as the new ventilator settings after repeating a briefer lung recruiting maneuver (1-2 minutes). This approach to setting PIP and PEEP can be done manually, but some ventilators have a special trending monitoring mode (as seen in Figure 5-5) to simplify the procedure. Clinical results of lung recruitment maneuvers have shown varied success but may indicate the technique works best on early stage ARDS patients.

OVERDISTENSION

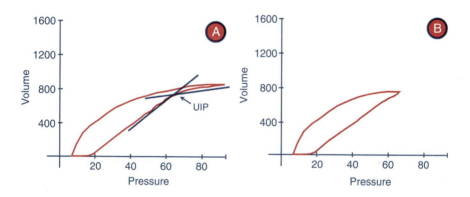

Figure 5-6. Identification and correction of overdistension as seen in P-V loops. (UIP = upper inflection point)

Overdistension occurs when the volume capacity of the lungs has been exceeded and the application of additional pressure causes very little increase in volume (loop A in Figure 5-5). The volume limit is identified on the P-V loop as an abrupt change in compliance in the terminal portion of inspiration, a second inspiratory inflection point (upper inflection point). This abnormal loop shape is commonly termed *beaking* and results in a reduced slope having a decreased dynamic compliance. Overdistension can lead to volutrauma and biotrauma (release of inflammatory mediators), particularly in lung regions with normal alveoli. Correction of overdistension involves decreasing the pressure setting in pressure-targeted ventilation or decreasing the volume setting in volume-targeted ventilation. The loop in graph B shows that a small decrease in the set tidal volume produced a large decrease in the PIP.

ACTIVE EXHALATION

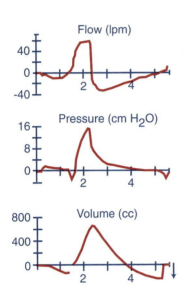

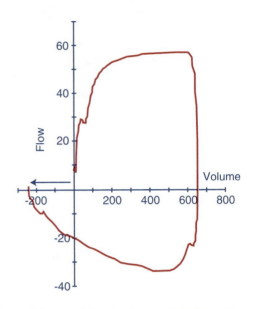

Figure 5-7. Active exhalation displayed in scalars.

Figure 5-8. Active exhalation displayed in F-V loop.

When a patient exhales more than the inspiratory volume, active exhalation has occurred. The waveforms in Figures 5-7, 5-8, and 5-9 show active exhalation of an additional volume of about 200 mL. For expiratory volume to be greater than inspiratory volume, the patient has to exhale below FRC. It is normal for this to happen occasionally in the clinical setting, for example, when the patient changes position, experiences a twinge of pain, or tries to cough. It is not normal if it happens in a regular pattern. Patients with air-trapping will often show a pattern of an active exhalation occurring every few breaths in attempt to relieve the trapped volume. A larger expiratory volume than inspiratory volume on every breath indicates the expiratory flow transducer is out of calibration or some other equipment error exists.

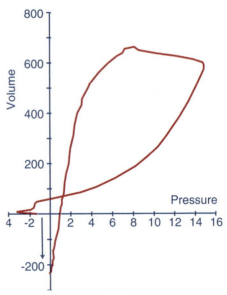

Figure 5-9. Active exhalation displayed in P-V loop.

BRONCHOSPASM: BRONCHODILATOR BENEFIT ASSESSMENT

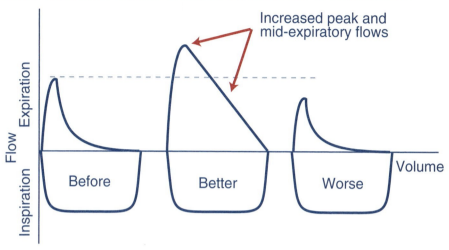

Figure 5-10. Indicators of airway improvement in the F-V loop as a result of response to a bronchodilator.

The effects of a bronchodilator are best appreciated in the F-V loop (Figure 5-10). The two major changes that indicate improvement are an increased peak expiratory flow rate and an increased mid-expiratory flow rate. Decreased mid-expiratory flow rates produce a scooped appearance in the descending portion of the expiratory curve (the Before and Worse loops in Figure 5-10). An improvement from bronchodilator will yield an increased tidal volume in pressure-targeted ventilation and sometimes in volume-targeted ventilation. An example of a positive bronchodilator response is given in Figure 5-11. Loop B shows increased peak and mid-expiratory flow rates compared to the pretreatment loop A.

Response to bronchodilator can also be seen in P-V loops. Loop B in Figure 5-12 shows decreased loop hysteresis compared to loop A. The maximal volume is slightly increased in this volume-targeted breath. Pressure-targeted ventilation tends to show similar and often more pronounced pre- and post-bronchodilator changes in the P-V loop given the same lung conditions. It is very useful to store a pre- and post-bronchodilator F-V loop in computer memory or print them for comparison. Comparing pre- and post-bronchodilator loops in one's memory is unreliable. It is best to keep the same axis scaling for both measurements if possible for ease of comparison.

Lack of response to bronchodilator may indicate that increased airways resistance is not due to bronchospasm. Airway narrowing may be due to fluid in the airways or swelling of the mucosa due to an inflammatory process not responsive to beta$_2$ agonists, or parasympatholytic agents. Pre- and post-loops after a trial of steroids may be

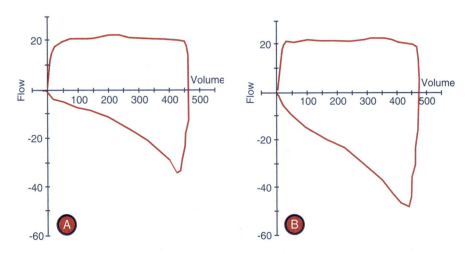

Figure 5-11. Pre- and post-bronchodilator F-V loops of volume-targeted breaths.

helpful for guiding therapy. Pre- and post loops can also be used for assessing which type of bronchodilator works best for a particular patient or if some combination of drugs has a superior effect. A post-drug loop that is worse than the pre-drug loop may indicate the patient is reacting to the drug propellent or preservative.

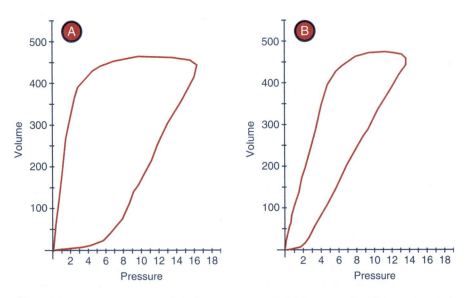

Figure 5-12. Pre- and post-bronchodilator P-V loops of volume-targeted breaths.

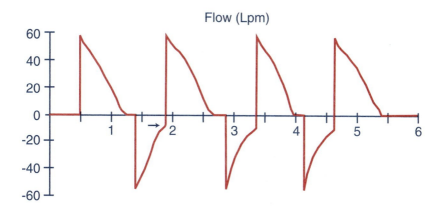

Figure 5-13. Flow scalar showing air-trapping due to dynamic hyperinflation.

Air-trapping and the associated auto-PEEP is generally caused by two mechanisms: dynamic hyperinflation and early collapse of unstable airways during exhalation. Dynamic hyperinflation occurs when the respiratory rate does not allow sufficient time for complete exhalation before the next breath. Figure 5-13 demonstrates this condition with early termination of exhalation indicated by the arrow. A similar example of early termination of exhalation is shown in the F-V loop of Figure 5-14. If dynamic hyperinflation is due to an excessive patient triggered respiratory rate it

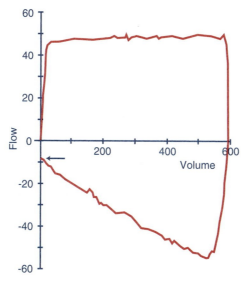

Figure 5-14. Air-trapping identified in the F-V loop of a volume-targeted breath.

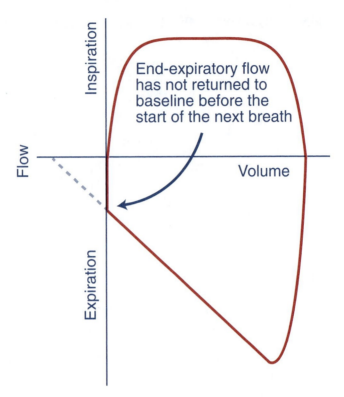

Figure 5-15. Conceptual illustration of why the F-V loop is altered by air-trapping.

may be helpful to switch to SIMV mode or, if necessary, sedate the patient. If a high respiratory rate is necessary and dynamic hyperinflation occurs, especially when bronchospasm is also present, increasing the inspiratory flow rate may yield improvement by extending the time for exhalation.

To better understand why the F-V loop changes shape at the end of exhalation, a conceptualized rendering is given in Figure 5-15. If expiratory time was extended the loop would follow the path of the light blue dashed line. Instead, the loop returns abruptly to the baseline at the start of the next breath. The potential additional volume is exaggerated in this example to clarify the concept of air-trapping. It is important to note that these examples only detect the presence of air-trapping and do not quantify it in cm H_2O.

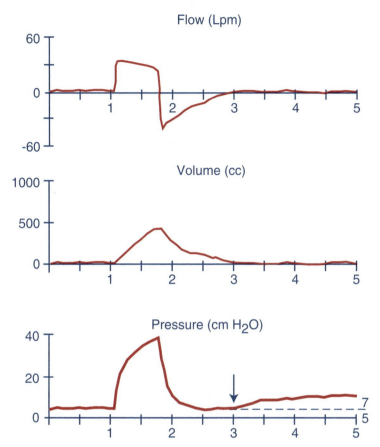

Figure 5-16. Measurement of auto-PEEP in a patient with early airways collapse during expiration. (Set PEEP of 5 cm H_2O, auto-PEEP of 7 cm H_2O, total of 12 cm H_2O.)

The other cause of air-trapping relates to the early collapse of small airways during expiration. Lung diseases that cause destruction of normal airway structure result in tissue being replaced by scar tissue that collapses more easily. This results in early airway closure during expiration. Auto-PEEP associated with air-trapping can be measured by using either of two clinical techniques. The dynamic technique requires the simultaneous measurement of esophageal pressure and will not be addressed here. The second technique involves measuring the airway pressure while occluding the expiratory side of the ventilator circuit near end exhalation (Figure 5-16). The end expiratory occlusion technique for measuring auto-PEEP requires sufficient expiratory time for the occlusion pressure to reach a plateau or the value will not be accurate. Patient respiratory efforts during the expiratory occlusion will also interfere with accurate measurements.

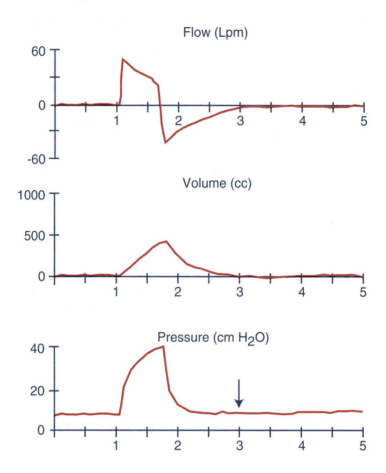

Figure 5-17. Application of external PEEP to correct auto-PEEP caused by early airways collapse during expiration.

The end expiratory occlusion technique is displayed in Figure 5-16. The arrow indicates the occlusion of the expiratory circuit after the end of the expiratory time. The airway pressure tracing rises and eventually plateaus at a level of 14 cm H_2O. This represents 5 cm H_2O of PEEP and 7 cm H_2O of auto-PEEP. Correction of this auto-PEEP is attempted in Figure 5-17. The external PEEP was increased to 8 cm H_2O in this case because the patient was known to have early small airway collapse (as in emphysema). The end expiratory occlusion measurement now indicates an acceptable 2 cm H_2O of auto-PEEP (total of 10 cm H_2O). Other causes of auto-PEEP should be addressed by other remedies such as increasing inspiratory flow, decreasing minute ventilation by frequency and/or V_T, bronchodilators, etc.

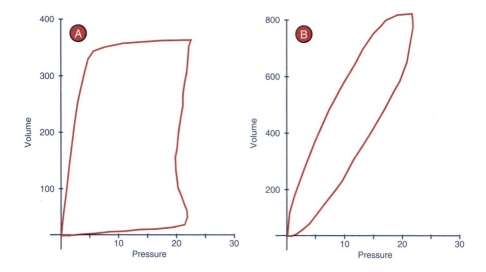

Figure 5-18. The effect of a kinked endotracheal tube on the P-V loop during pressure-targeted ventilation.

A kinked endotracheal tube (ETT) can occur suddenly or gradually. When passing a suction catheter through the ETT becomes difficult, the possibility of a partially obstructed ETT should be considered. This condition is a type of upper airway obstruction, shown in loop A of Figure 5-18. Note the considerable hysteresis and low tidal volume associated with a PIP of 22 cm H_2O. Attempts to reposition the ETT and the patient's head were unsuccessful at relieving the obstruction because a memory of bend in the tubing had developed. Loop B shows the resolution of the obstruction after replacement of the ETT. Partial obstruction of an artificial airway can also be caused by dried secretions or blood in the lumen or at the end of the tube.

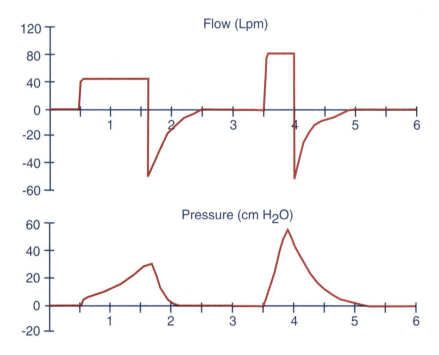

Figure 5-19. Dyssynchrony due to flow starvation.

Setting the inspiratory flow rate optimally in volume-targeted ventilation is often overlooked. This simple adjustment can improve patient comfort in general and especially when resting a patient on the ventilator who is being weaned by increasing periods of spontaneous breathing. The pressure scalar of the first breath in Figure 5-19 shows flow starvation or inadequate flow, a concave or downward scooped pressure curve during the inspiratory phase. The peak flow rate was increased in the second breath to better match the patient's inspiratory demand. Increasing the peak flow worked in this example, but setting the flow too high can produce turbulence that may lead to pressure limiting.

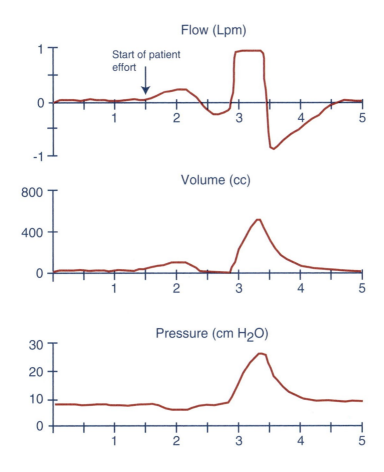

Figure 5-20. Failure to trigger a machine breath in response to patient inspiratory efforts due to an inappropriate sensitivity setting.

The three scalars in Figure 5-20 all show signs of patient effort around the two second time mark, but no machine breath was triggered. Although the pressure drop due to the patient's effort was not large, it was sustained for nearly a second. The patient's diaphragmatic strength may be marginal. Continued unsatisfied patient efforts can lead to patient anxiety further compromising of the diaphragm.

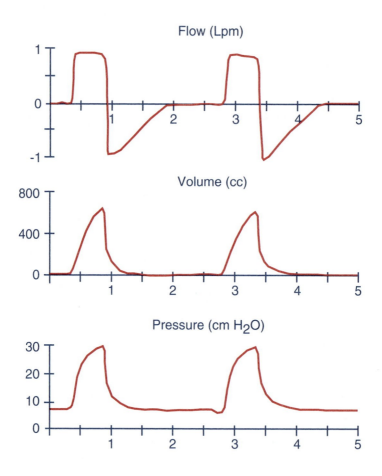

Figure 5-21. Ventilator sensitivity increased to allow for ventilator response to patient inspiratory efforts.

The first breath in Figure 5-21 was untriggered, indicated by the lack of pressure or flow change immediately prior to the machine breath. The second breath is an assisted breath as indicated by the slight pressure deflection before the machine breath. The sensitivity has been increased so that a machine breath is triggered before the patient can generate the magnitude of spontaneous effort observed in Figure 5-20.

PATIENT AND VENTILATOR RATES OUT OF SYNCHRONY

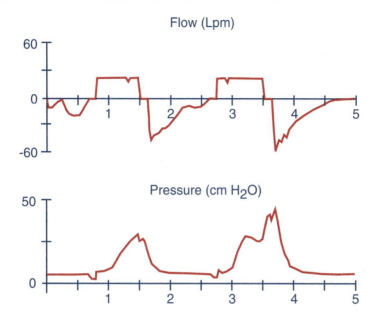

Figure 5-22. Patient rate and ventilator rate out of synchrony.

Patient ventilator rate dyssynchony can have several causes. A patient may have a very high spontaneous rate due to a sensation of air hunger or as a result of a neurologic injury. Aside from the acid base and air-trapping problems that can occur from supporting a high respiratory rate, if compliance and resistance are normal the machine breaths may remain synchronous with the patient up to a point. Beyond that point, patient and machine patterns become uncoupled. Patients with neurologic injury can become uncoupled from the ventilator pattern even at normal spontaneous rates.

Clinicians sometimes confuse rate dyssnychrony with flow starvation (Figure 5-19). Unlike flow starvation, the scalars in Figure 5-22 show abnormal patterns in the expiratory phase as well as the inspiratory phase. Also, the abnormal pattern changes from breath to breath, whereas the pattern for flow starvation is typically similar for each breath.

Choosing a ventilatory mode with rapid initial delivery such as PCV with PSV can often help minimize this type dyssynchrony. Fine-tuning the ventilator to the patient in this fashion will hopefully decrease the need for patient sedation. Some patients requiring full ventilatory support are difficult to synchronize even with using PCV and may respond best to just PSV. The pressure level can be titrated to best match the patient's pattern within the range needed for adequate gas exchange. Apnea ventilation parameters must be properly set before attempting such a trial.

LEAKS

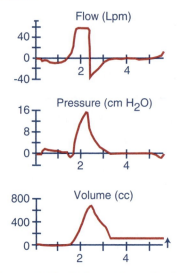

Figure 5-23. Volume loss displayed in a volume scalar.

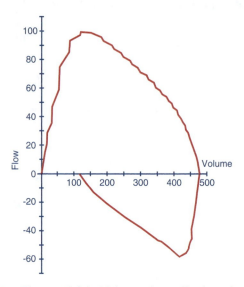

Figure 5-24. Volume loss displayed in a F-V loop.

Volume leaks can be easily detected in the volume scalar, F-V loop, and P-V loop. The volume scalar of Figure 5-23 does not return to the baseline during exhalation for the displayed breath. A plateau above the zero volume baseline is created by the lost volume (arrow). Volume loss is detected in the F-V and P-V loops as a failure to close the loops (Figures 5-24 and 5-25). Inspiratory and expiratory volume should be the same but will vary slightly even under normal conditions due to momentary changes in patient lung conditions, cuff seal, etc. Consistent volume loss should be systematically investigated for correction. A source of leak that is sometimes hard to identify is a misplaced nasogastric tube in the trachea, especially if one is unaware the tube has been replaced. In this situation, expiratory volume loss is accompanied by the patient exerting greater effort to trigger a ventilator breath.

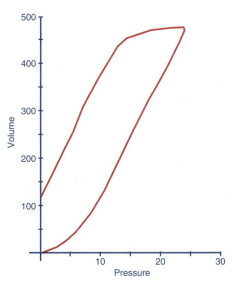

Figure 5-25. Volume loss displayed in a P-V loop.

CHAPTER 6
NEONATAL APPLICATIONS

I.   Introduction
II.   Normal Infant Pulmonary Functions
III.   Normal Scalars, Flow-Volume (F-V), and Pressure-Volume (P-V)
        Loops
IV.   Abnormal Waveforms
                Improper Sensitivity Scalars
                Large Air Leak and Autocycling Scalars
                A/C Pressure Control Asychrony Scalars
                A/C Pressure Control F-V and P-V Loops
        Inadequate Flow Scalars
                Inadequate Rise Time or Flow
                Excessive Inspiratory Pressure and Flow Scalars
                Effect of Excessive Inspiratory Pressure on the
                P-V Loop
                Reduced Compliance F-V and P-V Loops
                Excessive Inspiratory Time Scalars
        Inspiratory Flow Termination Scalars
                Termination of Inspiratory Flow
                Breath-Stacking (Auto-PEEP) Scalars
                Breath-Stacking F-V and P-V Loops
                Obstruction to Expiratory Flow Scalars
                Obstruction to Expiratory F-V and P-V Loops
                Right Mainstem Intubation Scalars
                Right Mainstem Intubation F-V and P-V Loops
                Progression to Extubation Scalars
                Turbulent Baseline Flow Rate Scalars
                High Frequency Ventilation

INTRODUCTION

Mechanical ventilation of neonates and small infants is commonly applied by a time triggered, pressure limited, time cycled ventilator. These ventilators have a continuous flow that delivers a specific F_1O_2. During spontaneous breathing, the continuous flow provides a fresh gas source to the patient. Mandatory or controlled breaths are based on setting of the inspiratory time (time cycled) and frequency (time triggered). When the ventilator time triggers a breath a signal is sent to the exhalation valve to close. Flow (decelerating flow curve) enters the patient's lungs through the inspiratory limb of the patient circuit for the set inspiratory time. When pressure reaches the set limit, the remaining pressure is diverted to a limiting device. As the ventilator cycles the exhalation valve opens and allows the patient volume and continuous flow to exit. Tidal volume delivered by the ventilator depends on the pressure limit, inspiratory time and flow rate. The amount of volume entering the lungs depends on lung and chest wall compliance, resistance of the endotracheal tube, and airways.

Over the past several years, neonatal ventilation has become more sophisticated. The first step was the adaptation of well established modes of adult ventilation into the Neonatal Intensive Care Unit (NICU) environment, such as synchronize intermittent mandatory ventilation (SIMV) and synchronized assist control as well as the ability to monitor bedside respiratory mechanics. Due to more recent technological advances, ventilators with sophisticated modes and features which had been reserved for use in the adult intensive care unit are frequently utilized in the NICU. Pressure control ventilation (PVC) and pressure support ventilation (PSV) with decelerating flow rates controlled by the ventilator are now an option. Volume-targeted ventilation is now possible as we are no longer limited to only pressure-targeted ventilation. Breath initiation and breath termination can be adjusted to more closely suit each individual patient's needs. As more ventilator modes and options become available to the clinician, the ability to monitor and assess through ventilator graphics becomes an even more valuable and essential tool.

The benefits of bedside respiratory monitoring include recognition of:
a. Asynchronous breathing
b. Breath-stacking, air-trapping and auto-PEEP
c. Expiratory grunting, prolong expiratory time
d. Change in dynamic compliance from lung disease or administration of surfactant
e. Inadvertent extubation
f. Excessive inspiratory pressure
g. Inappropriate inspiratory flow rate
h. Inappropriate sensitivity setting
i. Excessive inspiratory time
j. Excessive inspiratory flow rate
k. Excessive endotracheal tube leak
l. Identification of airway obstruction and the need for suctioning

NORMAL INFANT PULMONARY FUNCTIONS

Measurement	Units	Normal	RDS	BPD
Tidal volume	mL/kg	5-7	4-6	4-7
Respiratory rate	breaths/min	30-60	50-80	45-80
Minute ventilation	mL/kg/min	200-300	250-400	200-400
Function residual capacity (FRC)	mL/kg	20-30	15-20	20-30
Compliance (static)	mL/cm H_2O/kg	1-4	0.1-0.6	0.2-0.8
Compliance (dynamic)	mL/cm H_2O/kg	1-2	0.3-0.5	0.2-0.8
Resistance	cm H_2O/mL/sec	0.025-0.05	0.06-.15	0.03-0.15
Resistance	cm H_2O/L/sec	25-50	60-150	30-150
Work-of-breathing	gram/cm/min/kg	500-1000	800-3000	1800-6500
VD/VT ratio	percent	22-38	60-80	35-60
Dead space	mL/kg	1.0-2.0	3.0-4.5	3.0-4.5
Pulmonary capillary blood flow	mL/kg/min	160-230	75-140	120-200
Oxygen consumption	mL/kg/min	6-8		
CO_2 production	mL/kg/min	5-6		
Respiratory quotient		0.75-0.83		
Calories	kcal/kg/day	105-183		

(Adapted from SensorMedics Corporation, Yorba Linda, California)

NORMAL SCALARS, FLOW-VOLUME (F-V), AND PRESSURE-VOLUME (P-V) LOOPS

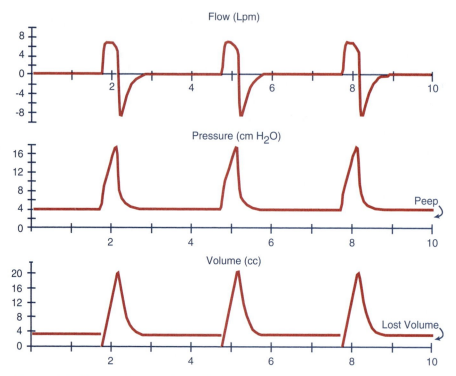

Figure 6-1. Neonatal control ventilation scalars.

The scalars in Figure 6-1 show mandatory or controlled breaths delivered by a time triggered, pressure limited, time cycled ventilator. The pressure scalar following a positive pressure breath (PPB) returns to baseline pressure of 4 cm H_2O representing PEEP. The driving pressure is 14 cm H_2O (18 cm H_2O - 4 cm H_2O = 14 cm H_2O). These breaths being mandatory breaths show no drop in pressure below baseline that would indicate a spontaneous inspiratory effort by the patient.

The flow scalar shows a flow rate of 8 L/m with a decelerating flow. The exhalation portion of the flow curve returns to baseline before the next breath is delivered. The volume scalar returns to baseline of 3 mL indicating lost volume. This is normal for a patient with a cuffless endotracheal tube where some volume leaks around the tube as a PPB is delivered to the lungs. Lost volume should not exceed 20% of the total volume delivered. Lost volume here represents 15%.

The F-V loop in Figure 6-2 shows a flow rate of 8 L/min and a delivered volume of 20 mL. The loop rises as flow rate enters the lung and a volume of 20 mL is achieved. That pressure is maintained for the set inspiratory time. When inspiratory time is complete, exhalation is represented by a downward loop. This corresponds to the flow scalar on the expiration side. The loop then returns to baseline. The return volume (exhalation portion of the loop) returns to 3 mL. This represents lost volume that corresponds to the volume scalar.

The P-V loop in Figure 6-3 shows a pressure of 18 cm H_2O (driving pressure is 14 cm H_2O) delivery and an exhaled volume of 17 mL (20 mL – 3 mL). The P-V loop starts at 4 cm H_2O representing the level of PEEP set on the ventilator.

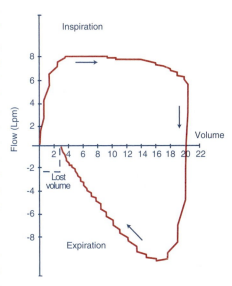

Figure 6-2. Control ventilation F-V loop.

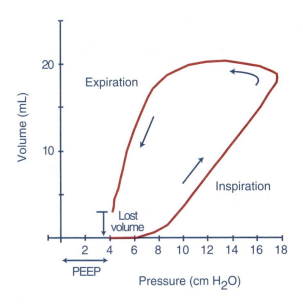

Figure 6-3. Control ventilation P-V loop.

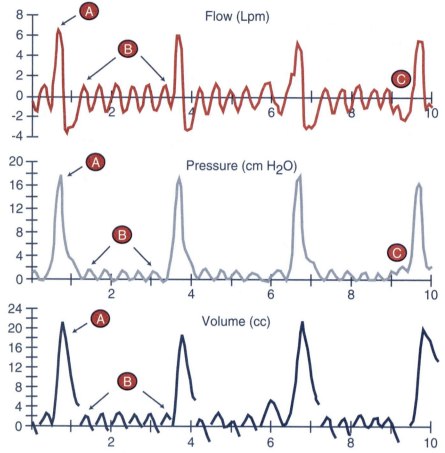

Figure 6-4. IMV scalars.

A patient is receiving pressure limited, time cycled, continuous flow ventilation in intermittent mandatory ventilation (IMV) mode (Figure 6-4). Point A represents a positive pressure breathing, and B represents spontaneous breaths on the flow, pressure, and volume scalar. The first three positive pressure breaths are delivered in synchronous with the patient's inspiratory effort. At point C, the patient begins to exhale but before complete exhalation occurs a positive pressure breath is delivered. Compare this with SIMV scalars in Figure 6-7.

Figure 6-5 shows F-V loops for the segment of breathing shown in Figure 6-4. The mandatory machine breaths are shown in red and blue, and spontaneous breaths are represented in light blue. Because the ventilator in this example used a simple interruption of constant flow to generate breaths, the machine breaths were susceptible to slight alterations by the patient's respiratory efforts.

The P-V loops for respirations in Figure 6-4 are given in Figure 6-6. Note the change in volumes as patient compliance changes from breath to breath.

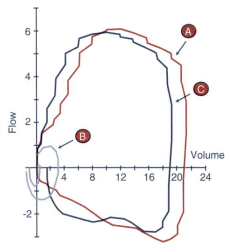

Figure 6-5. IMV F-V loops.

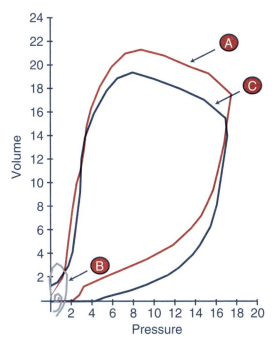

Figure 6-6. IMV P-V loops.

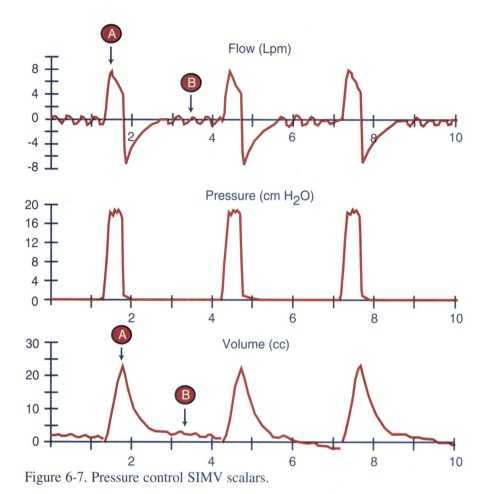

Figure 6-7. Pressure control SIMV scalars.

The patient in Figure 6-7 is receiving pressure-targeted ventilation in the SIMV mode. Point A represents a positive pressure breath. Point B represents spontaneous breaths. Note that at the end of each series of spontaneous breaths, the next positive pressure breath is delivered at end exhalation as seen on the flow scalar as the exhalation portion of the flow curve returns (resets) to baseline.

The F-V loops in Figure 6-8 were created with a ventilator in a pressure-targeted mode synchronized with the patient's inspiratory efforts, which yielded more uniform machine breaths. Although the volume was fairly constant in the example, it can vary according to amount of patient effort in a pressure-targeted mode.

The machine P-V loops in Figure 6-9 clearly indicate a pressure-targeted mode is being used. Inspiratory pressure quickly increases to the set limit and is maintained until the end of the inspiratory period.

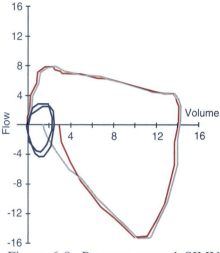

Figure 6-8. Pressure control SIMV F-V loops.

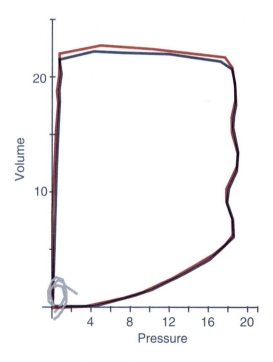

Figure 6-9. Pressure control SIMV P-V loops.

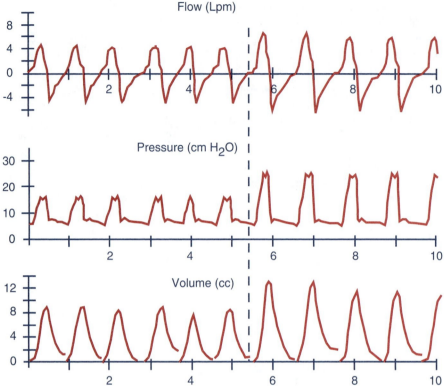

Figure 6-10. Pressure support ventilation of 10-20 cm H_2O with CPAP of 5 cm H_2O scalars.

The scalars in Figure 6-10 represent a change in PSV from 10-20 cm H_2O with a baseline CPAP of 5 cm H_2O. A PSV level of 10 cm H_2O with a baseline of 5 cm H_2O yields a total pressure of 15 cm H_2O with a driving pressure of 10 cm H_2O (15 cm H_2O - 5 cm H_2O = 10 cm H_2O). When PSV level is increased to 20 cm H_2O, flow and volume increase due to the increase in driving pressure to 20 cm H_2O (25 cm H_2O - 5 cm H_2O = 20 cm H_2O).

IMPROPER SENSITIVITY SCALARS

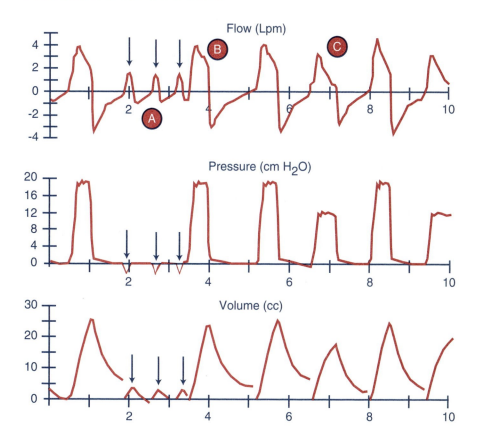

Figure 6-11. Improper sensitivity setting scalars.

The patient in Figure 6-11 is in SIMV mode with PSV. The flow, pressure, and volume scalars indicate spontaneous breaths at point A. Each arrow represents a spontaneous breath. Note on the pressure scalar there are negative pressure deflections that are not followed with a delivered pressure support breath. The sensitivity of the ventilator is improper for the inspiratory effort of the infant. Point B represents delivery of a positive pressure breath after which the sensitivity was increased. Point C represents a PS breath being delivered as a result of the new sensitivity setting.

LARGE AIR LEAK AND AUTOCYCLING SCALARS

Air leaks can have a variety of causes. They can be either mechanical in origin, such as a leak in a ventilator circuit, around a patient's endotracheal tube, or a large chest tube leak. They can also be of a patient origin, such as a bronchopleural fistula. Uncuffed endotracheal tubes are routinely used in the Neonatal and Pediatric ICU, therefore an endotracheal tube leak is the most common situation causing an air leak in children. A small leak is usually very manageable for a skilled clinician, but a large leak can be very problematic. In an air leak situation, the ventilator may not adequately maintain the baseline PEEP. The ventilator may inaccurately sense the PEEP baseline drift as a patient effort and respond with a supported breath. This is called autocycling. Some of the dangers of autocycling include air-trapping, auto-PEEP, asynchrony, hyperventilation, and delayed ventilator weaning. Large air leaks may also lead to a poor ventilator response to true patient respiratory efforts leading to an increase in the work-of-breathing and patient agitation.

Some of the signs you may observe on the scalar graphics that may demonstrate the presence of a large air leak include the inability to maintain PEEP on the pressure scalar, the presence of supported breaths without an obvious trigger such a pressure or flow change, and the tidal volume scalar not returning to baseline as demonstrated in Figure 6-12.

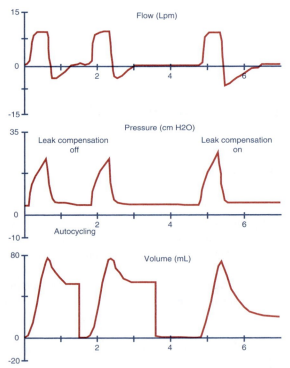

Figure 6-12. Large air leak and autocycling scalars.

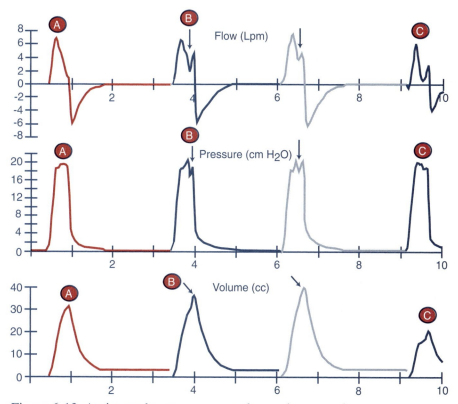

Figure 6-13. Assist mode pressure control asynchrony scalars.

The first breath A on the flow, pressure, and volume scalars represents normal synchronous breathing (Figure 6-13). Compare these waveforms to the next three waveforms on each scalar. On the flow scalar, arrows pointing to the notched area during inspiratory phase indicates an inspiratory effort. Fluctuation in pressure occurs during the inspiratory effort as seen on the pressure scalar. This coincides with fluctuation in flow as the infant inspires. The volume scalar demonstrates fluctuation in volume. The second and third volume waveforms show increases in volume as a result of the inspiration taken during the positive pressure breath. The third volume waveform shows a reduction due to asynchrony. To improve synchrony the clinician could either shorten inspiratory time or increase inpiratory pressure.

ASSIST MODE PRESSURE CONTROL ASYNCHRONY F-V AND P-V LOOPS

The loops and numbers in Figures 6-14 and 6-15 correspond with those in Figure 6-13. Inspiratory flow normally follows a decreasing pattern after reaching a peak flow (red loop). Figure 6-14 shows flow increasing and decreasing twice during the inspiratory phase due to patient-ventilator asynchrony (blue and light blue loops). Asynchrony is seen where flow is decreasing and then an upswing in the flow-volume curve occurs. This is due to the patient initiating another inspiratory effort near the end of the ventilator's inspiratory period. Note the alteration in volume with each breath.

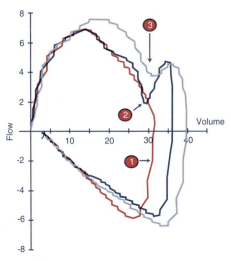

Figure 6-14. Assist mode pressure control asynchrony F-V loops.

The P-V loops in Figure 6-15 show a rapid initial rise in pressure as volume enters the lung. Change in the loop occurs as the infant inspires during the inspiratory phase of the positive pressure breath. Each P-V loop can be compared to the scalars in Figure 6-13. Note the change in volume of each P-V loop from 1 to 2, and 2 to 3. The continual rise in pressure to the set point indicates flow is adequate for the patient (red loop).

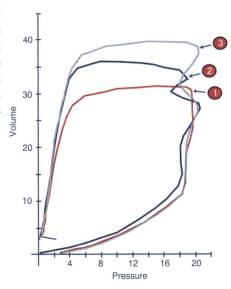

Figure 6-15. Assist mode pressure control asynchrony P-V loops.

INADEQUATE FLOW SCALARS

INADEQUATE RISE TIME OR FLOW

In some ventilator modes, the flow at the onset of inspiration phase can be determined by the setting of the rise time. The rise time is the time required to reach the set pressure level. The rise time is clinician adjusted and is often utilized to improve patient comfort. Rapid rise time may decrease the patient's work-of-breathing, the feeling of dyspnea, and the need for sedatives. Rise times that are either too fast or too slow may be detrimental. Flow rates that are too fast may prematurely terminate the inspiratory phase of a breath, since some breath termination criteria utilize a calculation based on a percentage of the peak flow. High flow rates may also potentially activate an inspiratory termination reflex, resulting in brief, shallow respirations. Flow rates that are too slow may cause flow starvation and dyssynchrony, increased work-of-breathing, inadequate mean airway pressure, and lead to the increase of peak airway pressure to attain tidal volumes.

Inadequate rise time produces inadequate flow for the patient as illustrated in the pressure and flow scalars of Figure 6-16.

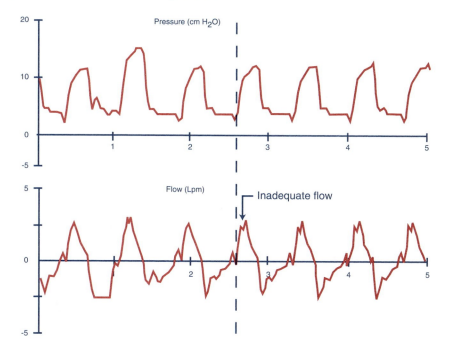

Figure 6-16. Inadequate flow scalars.

EXCESSIVE INSPIRATORY PRESSURE AND FLOW SCALARS

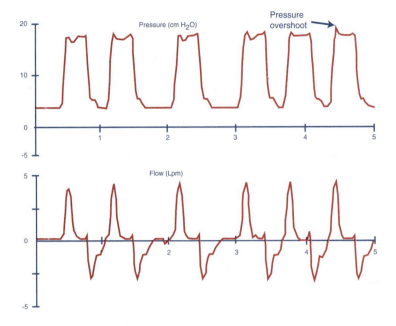

Figure 6-17. Excessive inspiratory pressure and flow scalars.

Excessive flow delivery can be caused by a rise time that is too fast. In the pressure scalar in Figure 6-17, an assist mode pressure control breath is delivered with the fastest rise time; notice the spike on the pressure scalar at the beginning of inspiration. Often this pressure spike is undesirable as it brings flow and pressure to the patient that does not translate into increased tidal volume delivery.

EFFECT OF EXCESSIVE INSPIRATORY PRESSURE ON THE P-V LOOP

Point A on the P-V curve in Figure 6-18 shows an increase in pressure with no change in volume. This is often referred to as *beaking*. At point B the pressure is decreased from 29 cm H_2O to 25 cm H_2O and the curve has a more rounded appearance at peak inspiration. Although the pressure is reduced, there is little change in the delivered volume.

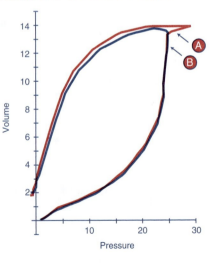

Figure 6-18. Effect of excessive inspiratory pressure on the P-V loop (beaking).

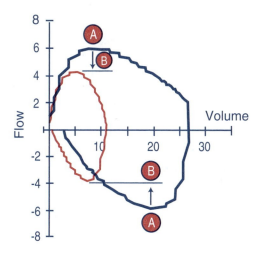

Figure 6-19. Reduced compliance F-V loop.

The F-V loop in Figure 6-19 represents a reduction in flow and volume as a result of decreased lung compliance. Loop A represents a high compliance with a 25 mL tidal volume being delivered. Loop B shows a reduction in compliance where tidal volume delivery is 10 mL. The P-V loop A in Figure 6-20 shows a similar volume as in the F-V loop A in Figure 6-19. Notice in loop B the flattening of the loop as compared to loop A, this indicates a compliance decrease.

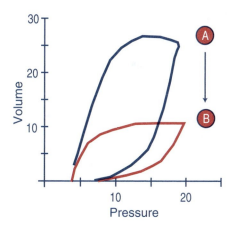

Figure 6-20. Reduced compliance P-V loop.

EXCESSIVE INSPIRATORY TIME SCALARS

Increased inspiratory time can be a valuable tool during the acute phase of the lung injury to increase mean airway pressure, treat atelectasis, and to improve oxygenation. As the lung recovers and the patient resumes spontaneous breathing, excessive inspiratory time can lead to active exhalation and dyssynchrony. Excessive inspiratory time can lead to patient agitation, increased carbon dioxide production, increased oxygen and caloric consumption, delayed ventilator weaning, increased intracranial pressure (ICP), increased risk of cerebral bleed, and a compromised cardiovascular status.

Excessive inspiratory time causes active exhalation as illustrated in the pressure and flow scalars in Figure 6-21. Notice the spiked appearance at the completion of each breath as the patient forcibly exhales due to an inspiratory time which is too long.

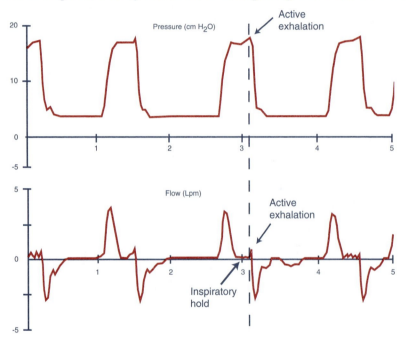

Figure 6-21. Excessive inspiratory time scalars.

TERMINATION OF INSPIRATORY FLOW SCALARS

A breath may be terminated by time or by flow. Flow termination facilitates synchrony by allowing the clinician to select the percent of peak flow at which inspiration terminates. Flow termination should be titrated by using graphics to eliminate periods of no inspiratory flow and of pressure plateau, but the patient's tidal volume should be preserved.

The addition of flow cycled termination instead of time cycled allows the transition from inspiration to expiration to occur, without a significant pressure plateau or zero flow state, as seen in the pressure and flow scalars in Figure 6-22. Notice the transition from peak inspiratory flow to peak expiratory flow is almost a straight line.

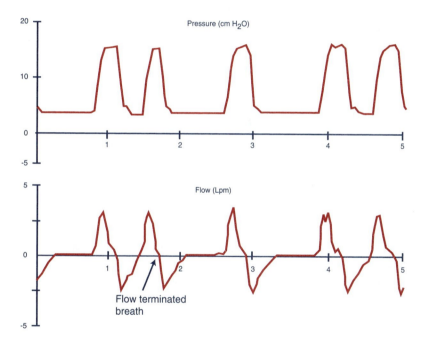

Figure 6-22. Inspiratory flow termination scalars.

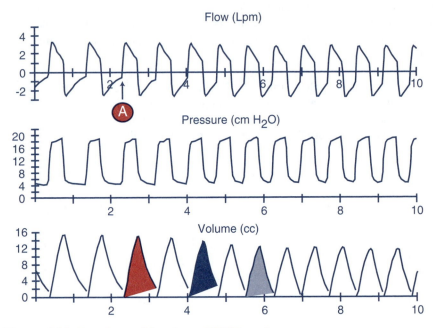

Figure 6-23. Breath-stacking (auto-PEEP) scalars.

A high mechanical ventilator rate can cause breath-stacking to occur, resulting in air-trapping or auto-PEEP. In Figure 6-23, note point A on the flow scalar how the flow does not reach baseline before the next mechanical breath is delivered. As the mechanical rate is changed (moving from left to right), note how the next positive pressure breath starts earlier. On the volume scalar, note how an increase in respiratory rate causes volume to decrease. Each new breath is stacked on top of the preceding breath causing air to remain trapped in the lung.

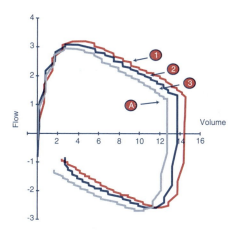

Figure 6-24. Breath-stacking F-V loops.

The F-V loops in Figure 6-24 labeled 1, 2, and 3 coincide with the shaded curves on the scalars in Figure 6-23. Note how each loop has a decrease in volume as the mechanical rate is increased and how flow does not reach baseline before the next positive pressure breath is delivered. The P-V loop in Figure 6-25 shows the volume retained in the lung at end exhalation. Also note how with each successive breath, the tidal volume decreases due to the trapped gas in the lung. Observe the large hysteresis created by breath-stacking.

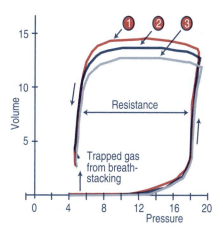

Figure 6-25. Breath-stacking P-V loops.

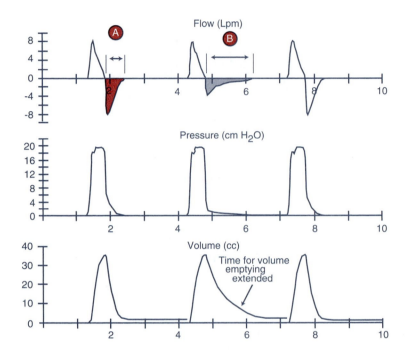

Figure 6-26. Obstruction to expiratory flow scalars.

Compare the shaded expiratory waveforms A and B in Figure 6-26. Waveform A shows a normal expiratory waveform reaching baseline in a short period of time. The expiratory waveform is a mirror image of the inspiratory waveform. In B, note how the expiratory waveform is shorter (less flow rate) and the expiratory time is longer. This indicates there is resistance to exhalation. Also note on the volume scalar the shape of the volume scalar as compared to the first volume scalar. The time for volume emptying is longer due to expiratory resistance. Also recognize how the volume baseline is raised compared to the first volume waveform. The second pressure waveform also shows extended time for emptying of the lung. No breath-stacking is seen here in spite of prolonged exhalation due to the long exhalation time set on the ventilator.

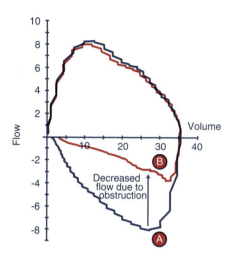

Figure 6-27. Expiratory flow rate obstruction F-V loops.

Compare points A and B in the F-V loop shown in Figure 6-27. The inspiratory flow is normal in both A and B. A decrease in expiratory flow rate occurs during grunting and less volume returns at B than at A. The P-V loop in Figure 6-28 shows a widened loop appearance from A to B, indicating a greater resistance, accompanied by expiratory grunting. The loop enlargement during exhalation indicates resistance during exhalation.

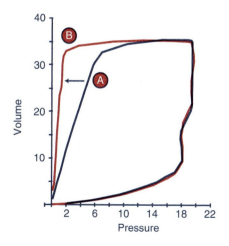

Figure 6-28. Expiratory flow rate obstruction P-V loops.

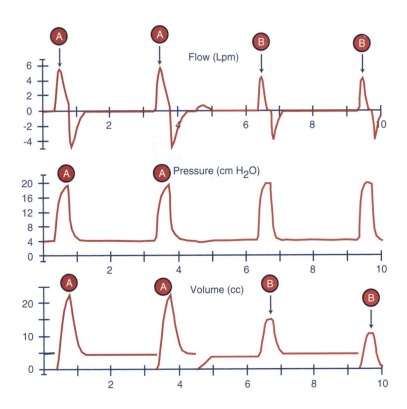

Figure 6-29. Neonatal right mainstem intubation scalars.

The scalars in Figure 6-29 show changes in flow rate and volume as the ET tube moves from the trachea into the right mainstem bronchus. Point A represents normal flow and volume and pressure scalars from proper placement of the ETT. Point B represents the tube having moved into the right mainstem bronchus. The volume scalar at point B shows a reduction in volume compared to point A and flow rate at point B is reduced compared to point A. Pressure remains unchanged in this pressure controlled mode of ventilation.

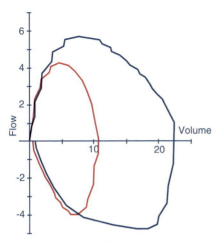

Right mainstem intubation results in a decreased volume and peak flow rate as seen in Figure 6-30. The red loop takes on the typical pattern for a restrictive condition. This is due to the decreased compliance of ventilating one lung.

A change in patient compliance during pressure-targeted ventilation causes change in both pressure and volume. The ventilator adjusts flow rate to maintain a constant pressure as seen in Figure 6-31. A change in patient respiratory system compliance using pressure-targeted ventilation results in a volume change.

Figure 6-30. Right mainstem bronchus intubation F-V loops.

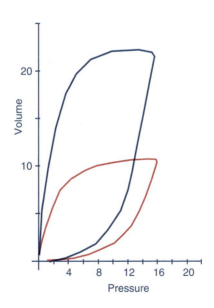

Figure 6-31. Right mainstem bronchus intubation P-V loops.

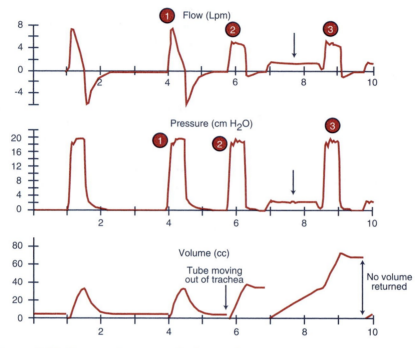

Figure 6-32. Progression to extubation scalars.

Breath 1 on the flow scalar in Figure 6-32 represents a normal condition with the ET tube positioned through the vocal cords into the trachea. Normal flow rate, pressure, and volume waveforms are seen at this point. As the tube starts to move out of the trachea, note the decrease in returned volumes. With the tube completely out of the trachea, no volume is returned. The flow and pressure curves are altered by the reduction in returned volume.

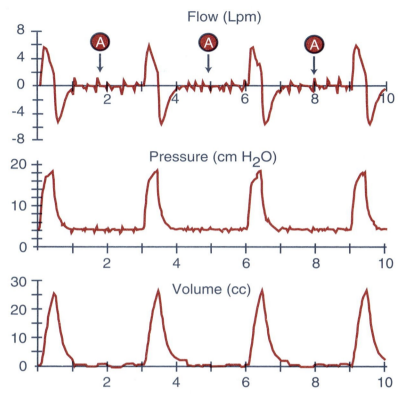

Figure 6-33. Turbulent baseline flow rate scalars.

Water from condensation in the inspiratory limb of the ventilator circuit creates nonuniform waveform appearance in each of the scalars between each positive pressure breath. This may also be caused by secretions in the endotracheal tube and airways or water within the inspiratory limb of the patient's circuit.

HIGH FREQUENCY VENTILATION

High frequency ventilation (HFV) is a mode of mechanical ventilation in which lung recruitment is accomplished without exposing the lungs to high peak pressures. Tidal volumes are utilized that are near dead space and the breaths are delivered at very high frequencies. The goals of HFV are to maintain a nearly constant alveolar volume and alveolar pressure to prevent lung stretch injuries. The main characteristics of high frequency ventilation are small tidal volumes, short inspiratory times, and optimally inflated alveoli. There are several different types of high frequency ventilators utilized in the United States and around the world. They all differ slightly in how the breaths are delivered, but the basic theory of operation is the same for all and the basic terms utilized to discuss their settings are closely related.

FACTORS AFFECTING GAS EXCHANGE

The following are the three main factors affecting gas exchange during HFV:

    a.   Frequency
    b.   Amplitude
    c.   Mean airway pressure

The measurement of the respiratory rate is called the frequency. Frequency is expressed in Hertz (Hz) or cycles per minute: one Hz = 60 cycles per minute.

For example, 10 Hz (10 x 60) = 600 cycles per minute.

Depending on the type of high frequency ventilator chosen, increasing the Hz, otherwise known as the frequency or respiratory rate, does not necessarily improve minute ventilation and gas exchange as in traditional modes of mechanical ventilation. In fact, the reverse actually occurs. In the most common form of HFV, a piston is used to push pulses of gas through a continuous flow circuit. Increasing the Hz or frequency in HFV can decrease the amount of time this piston spends in the inspiratory position (decreasing inspiratory time) which can decrease tidal volume delivered to the patient. To increase gas exchange in patients on HFV, often the Hz or frequency will be decreased not increased.

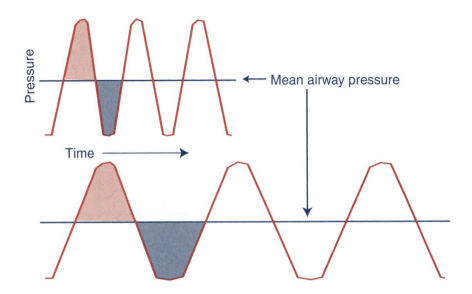

Figure 6-34. Frequency's affect on tidal volume displaced.

Frequency controls the time allowed (distance) for the piston to move. Therefore, the lower the frequency, the greater the volume displaced; the higher the frequency, the smaller the volume displaced. Increasing frequency in HFV with a piston driven ventilator will decrease tidal volume and minute ventilation and increase the patient's $PaCO_2$.

The amplitude adjustment affects the pulse volume or the amount of gas pushed back and forth through the circuit. The amplitude is not measured from baseline as PIP is above PEEP. Amplitude is a measurement of change above and below baseline. Increases in amplitude can increase tidal volume displacement and will directly affect ventilation. Amplitude adjustments are the first choice for the clinician who would like to increase or decrease carbon dioxide clearance in the patient on HFV.

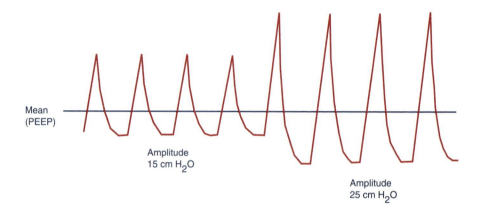

Figure 6-35. Amplitude is measured as the distance peak to trough from above and below the mean airway pressure.

The mean airway pressure adjustment is used to inflate the lung and to improve gas exchange, primarily oxygenation. The goal is to keep the alveoli above critical opening pressure and maintain them in the open position. With optimal lung expansion the alveoli may stabilize and be protected against overdistension and sheer stretch injuries.

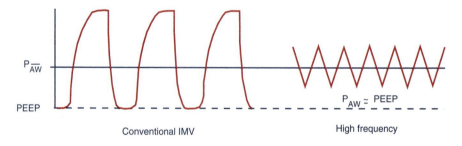

Figure 6-36. Mean airway pressure and PEEP are completely different measurements during conventional ventilation but the same during HFV.

NEONATAL CASE STUDY 1

A 20-year-old gave birth to Rodney, a 27-week, 785-gram baby born by vaginal delivery. The mother had no prenatal care, and she had premature rupture of membranes for three days prior to delivery. Apgar scores were 5 and 9 at 1 minute and 5 minutes, respectively, following bag-mask ventilation. Rodney was intubated with a 2.5 mm ID oral endotracheal tube and given one dose of surfactant. Rodney was transferred to NICU and placed on pressure limited, time cycled ventilation with the following settings: PIP 20 cm H_2O, rate 40/min, inspiratory time 0.3 seconds, PEEP 5 cm H_2O, F_IO_2 1.0. Ten hours after the initial dose of surfactant was given, Rodney exhibited signs of respiratory distress with intercostal and suprasternal retractions, spontaneous respiratory rate increased from 48 to 88/min, pulse increase from 138 to 178/min, and increased periods of desaturation below 90%. Exhaled tidal volume decreased from 5 mL/kg to 2.5 mL/kg. The F_IO_2, which had been weaned to 0.30, has been increased to 0.70 to maintain saturation above 90%. The following P-V curve B was obtained and compared to the P-V curve A taken after administration of the initial dose of surfactant.

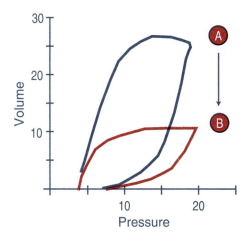

Figure A-1.

Questions

1.   What has caused the change in the P-V loop between A and B?

2.   Based on P-V loop B, what would you recommend at this time?

Answers to Neonatal Case Study 1

1. The P-V loop change from A to B indicates a decrease in lung compliance. Notice that the pressure remains the same at 20 cm H_2O, but the volume decreased from approximately 27 mL to 10 mL. Typically a reduced compliance causes a shift of the P-V loop to the right.

2. It would be appropriate to administer another dose of surfactant at this time in response to the reduced lung compliance.

NEONATAL CASE STUDY 2

Israel is a 27-week gestational age 800-gram infant born by vaginal delivery. The mother has just arrived from Mexico and has received no prenatal care. Israel is cyanotic and apneic at delivery with initial Apgars of 3 and 6 at 1 and 5 minutes. After initial bag and mask ventilation, he is intubated in the delivery room with a 2.5 mm endotracheal tube. Surfactant is immediately administered. He is transported to the NICU and placed on a time cycled, pressure limited, constant flow ventilator mode with the settings of SIMV of 36 breaths/minute, PIP of 13 cm H_2O, PEEP of 4 cm H_2O, inspiratory time of 0.4 seconds, and F_IO_2 of 0.70. His initial chest X-ray has an appearance consistent with respiratory distress syndrome. His initial ABG is 7.20, CO_2 of 55mmHg. PO_2 of 45mmHg, and BE of -5 mEq/L. His transcutaneous monitor is reading a CO_2 of 60 mm Hg and his oxygen saturation is 88%. Over the next several hours, Israel has repeated oxygen desaturations, the CO_2 measurement on his transcutaneous monitor is climbing, and he appears agitated. The following pressure and flow scalars are observed.

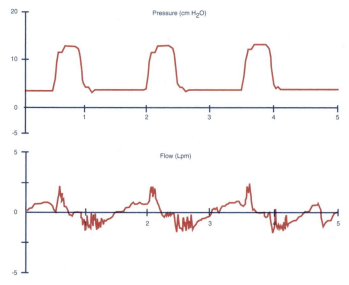

Figure A-2.

Questions

1.   What do these scalars indicate?

2.   What change was made at this time to improve this situation?

Answers to Neonatal Case Study 2

1.   These scalars indicate that Israel is in patient-ventilator asynchrony. Notice how he is making spontaneous inspiratory efforts at the end of each mechanical breath. There are negative pressure deflections on the pressure scalar at the end of inspiration and multiple flow changes on the flow scalar.

2.   Israel's ventilator mode was changed from SIMV with a constant flow pattern to PSV with a decelerating flow pattern. In PSV all of Israel's spontaneous efforts are supported and all his inspiratory flow demands are met. (See Figure A-3 below.)

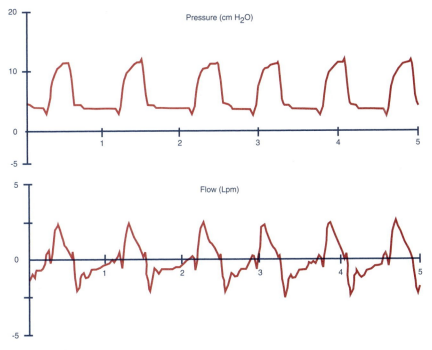

Figure A-3.

NEONATAL CASE STUDY 3

Vanessa is a 34-week estimated gestational age infant born Cesarean section. Her mother had excellent prenatal care, but Vanessa is delivered emergently due to abruptio placentae with Apgars of 4 and 6, at 1 and 5 minutes. After resuscitation in the delivery room, she is intubated with a 3.5 mm endotracheal tube and transported to the NICU. She is placed in an assist control pressure mode of ventilation with a PIP of 18 cm H_2O, PEEP of 3 cm H_2O, respiratory rate of 30/min, inspiratory time of 0.5 seconds, and an F_IO_2 1.0. Her chest X-ray initially shows streaky infiltrates radiating from the hilum of the lung and fluid within the interlobar tissue consistent with retained fetal lung fluid. Her initial ABG is 7.30, PCO_2 of 40 mm Hg, PO_2 of 50 mm Hg, and BE of -7 mEq/L. On day two, Vanessa appears agitated, her heart rate and CO_2 are elevated, and she is experiencing frequent oxygen desaturations. You observe the following pressure and flow scalar.

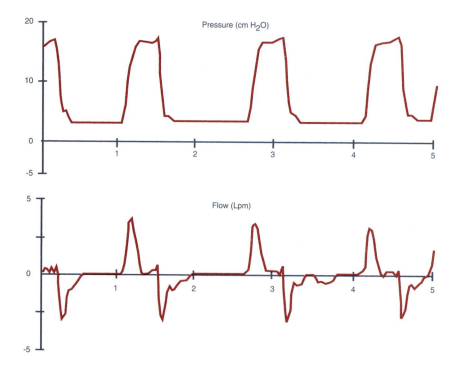

Figure A-4.

Questions

1.   What do these scalars indicate?

2.   What changes can be made to improve the situation?

Answers to Neonatal Case Study 3

1. The scalars illustrate excessive inspiratory time leading to active exhalation and dyssynchrony. Notice the spiked appearance at the completion of each breath as the patient forcibly exhales due to an inspiratory time which is too long. Increased inspiratory time can be a valuable tool to improve oxygenation. But as the lung recovers excessive inspiratory time can lead to patient agitation, increased carbon dioxide production, increased oxygen and caloric consumption, delayed ventilator weaning, and a compromised cardiovascular status.

2. To improve the situation the clinician can choose to cycle the breath with flow instead of time. Flow termination facilitates synchrony by allowing the clinician to select the percent of peak flow at which inspiration terminates to eliminate periods of no inspiratory flow and pressure plateau while maintaining the patient's tidal volume. Notice the transition from peak inspiratory flow to peak expiratory flow is now almost a straight line. (See Figure A-5 below.)

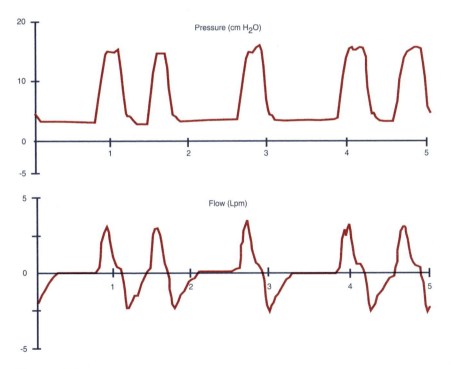

Figure A-5.

PEDIATRIC CASE STUDY 1

Austin is a 4-month old who was previously treated for RDS and BPD for three months which was the result of his immature birth at 28-weeks gestation. After being at home for just one month, Austin is brought to the Children's Hospital Emergency Department with what his mother reports as blue spells, coughing, gagging, large amounts of clear to white nasal secretions, poor feeding, and periods of apnea. Shortly after arriving in the ED, Austin stops breathing and is intubated with a 4.0 mm endotracheal tube. He is transported to the Pediatric Intensive Care Unit where he is placed on a mechanical ventilator in the assist control pressure mode with a slow rise time, PIP of 18 cm H_2O, PEEP of 4 cm H_2O, respiratory rate of 24 breaths/minute, and an F_IO_2 of .40. A chest X-ray is taken which shows perihilar infiltrates and right upper lobe atelectasis.

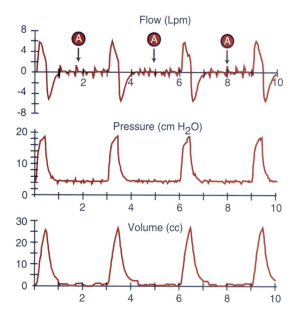

Figure A-6.

Questions

1.   What is abnormal about the flow, pressure, and tidal volume scalars for this patient?

2.   What should be done for this patient?

Answers to Pediatric Case Study 1

1. There is a nonuniform appearance on each scalar between every positive pressure breath. It is at the baseline of all three scalars. This can be caused by partial obstruction or water in the circuit anywhere between the ventilator and the patient.

2. This patient most likely requires airway suctioning. Also, check for condensation in the ventilator circuit.

ADULT CASE STUDY 1

Joyce is a 40-year-old black female, status post motor vehicle accident. After three days in the ICU she was being ventilated with volume-targeted SIMV at a V_T of 750 mL, PEEP of 7 cm H_2O, and set frequency of 16 breaths/minute.

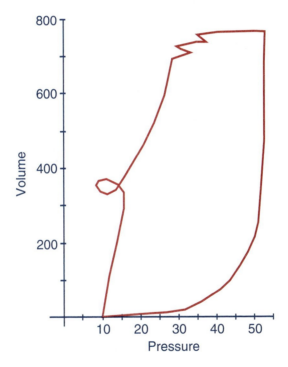

Figure A-7.

Questions

1. What is the dynamic compliance for this patient?

2. What abnormalities are present in the above P-V loop?

In an attempt to better synchronize the ventilator to the patient without sedation, the mode was changed to PSV with a set pressure of 28 cm H$_2$O. The resulting P-V loop is shown below.

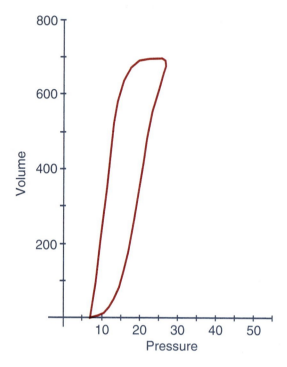

Figure A-8.

3.   What is the patient's dynamic compliance after the change?

4.   Would this ventilator change be considered an improvement or worsening of the patient's synchrony with the ventilator?

Answers to Adult Case Study 1

1.   The dynamic compliance was approximately 17 mL/cm H$_2$O.

2.   The P-V loop exhibited increased hysteresis, disruption/dyssynchrony at the beginning of exhalation, and a spontaneous inspiratory effort toward the end of exhalation.

3.   The dynamic compliance was approximately 33 mL/cm H$_2$O.

4.   For this particular patient, PSV mode improved patient-ventilator synchrony and yielded less loop hysteresis and improved compliance.

ADULT CASE STUDY 2

You have been working in the emergency department with a 45-year-old, female patient (height of 51 inches) in respiratory distress since the start of day shift. She arrived intubated and on a transport ventilator, but you were able to successfully switch her to PSV mode. Although she states that she prefers the PSV breaths, her breathing is clearly still not comfortable. The ventilator graphics display shows the waveforms on the left side of the figure below.

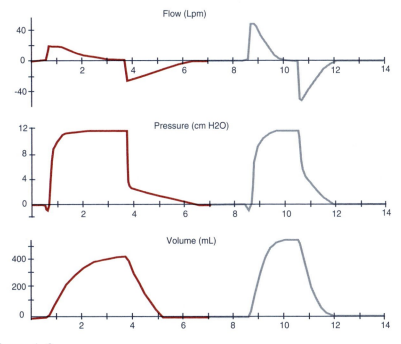

Figure A-9.

Questions

1.   What aspects of the graphic appear to be abnormal?

2.   Is the cause of these problems related to the ventilator settings or the patient's condition?

When you return to your patient on PSV after obtaining an arterial sample from another patient, a colleague informs you she was asked to attend to the patient in your absence. When you ask what she did for your patient she replied, "Not much besides retaping the ET tube." The graphics display now looks like the waveforms on the right side of the figure above.

3.   Did your colleague help or hinder the situation?

4.   What would you do now?

Answers to Adult Case Study 2

1.   The peak inspiratory flow was low (20 L/min) and the pressure plateau was extended (3 second inspiratory time, longer than normal).

2.   PSV breaths do not allow for setting the inspiratory flow; it is determined by patient variables. The inspiratory time is also under patient control. The tidal volume is a little less than desired for this patient's size, but note how the volume curves steadily increases despite the extended time at an inspiratory pressure plateau. A significant patient effort could produce this but would usually be accompanied by a large inspiratory flow rate and volume, which is not the case here. A decreased compliance could produce a decreased inspiratory flow but should also cause a rapid return to baseline for both the inspiratory and expiratory flows. The anomalies seen are consistent with a high resistance to flow.

3.   Something during the process of retaping the ET tube appears to have relieved much of the resistance problem. The inspiratory flow more than doubled and the tidal volume increased to more than 500 mL with a shorter inspiratory time. Perhaps a kink in the artificial airway was removed, the tip of the tube was moved away from the airway surface or pulled back above the carini, or some other aspect of obstruction to flow was reduced.

4.   Assess your patient for changes. Are there any remaining sources of airways resistance that could be reduced? Listen to breath sounds and check the ET tube position, patency, and if the size is appropriate for the patient. If a closed suction system is being used, is the catheter fully retracted?

APPENDIX B
VENT WAVEFORMS CHECKLIST

BIBLIOGRAPHY

The Acute Respiratory Distress Syndrome Network, "Ventilation with Lower Tidal Volumes as Compared with Traditional Tidal Volumes for Acute Lung Injury and the Acute Respiratory Distress Syndrome." *N Engl J Med 2000;* 342(18):1301-8.

Amato, M. Asia Pacific Association for Respiratory Care. Pressure support and pressure controlled ventilation: simple or complex modes? http://www.jichi.ac.jp/ aparc.japan/program/PCV & PSV-simple or comp15.doc. Accessed April 20, 2006.

Blanch, L. "Measurement of Air Trapping, Intrinsic Positive End-Expiratory Pressure, and Dynamic Hyperinflation in Mechanically Ventilated Patients." *Respiratory Care* 2005 Jan; 50(1):110-124.

Broseghini, C., et. al.: "Respiratory Resistance and Intrinsic Positive End-Expiratory Pressure (PEEP) in Patients with the Adult Respiratory Distress Syndrome (ARDS)." *Eur Respir J* 1988; 1:726-31.

Clinical Application of Mechanical Ventilation. 3rd ed. Albany: Delmar, 2006. (A student-friendly textbook on mechanical ventilation and related topics.)

Egan's Fundamentals of Respiratory Care. 8th ed. St. Louis: Mosby, 2003. (A comprehensive text on respiratory care including several chapters on mechanical ventilation and related topics.)

Henzler, D. et al. "Respiratory Compliance But Not Gas Exchange Correlates with Changes in Lung Aerations after a Recruitment Maneuver: An Experimental Study in Pigs with Saline Lavage Lung Injury." *Critical Care* 2005; 9: R471-82.

Hess, D.R., R.M. Kacmarek. *Essentials of Mechanical Ventilation.* 2nd ed. New York: McGraw-Hill, 2002. (A compact text designed for clinicians that provides quick reviews current practice in mechanical ventilation and supporting literature.)

Houston, P. "An Approach to Ventilation in Acute Respiratory Distress Syndrome." *Canadian Journal of Surgery* 43(4) 2000 Aug: 263-8.

Levy, M.M. "Optimal PEEP in ARDS. Changing Concepts and Current Controversies." *Critical Care Clinics* 2002; 18(1): 15-33.

Lim, S.C. et al. "Intercomparison of Recruitment Maneuver Efficacy in Three Models of Acute Lung Injury." *Critical Care Medicine* 2004; 32(12): 2371-2377.

Lu, Q., J.J. Rouby. "Measurement of Pressure-Volume Curves in Patients on Mechanical Ventilation: Methods and Significance." *Critical Care* 2000; 4(2): 91-100.

Lucangelo, U. "Respiratory Mechanics Derived from Signals in the Ventilator Circuit." *Respiratory Care 2005* Jan; 50(1): 55-67.

MacIntyre, N.R., R.D. Branson. *Mechanical Ventilation.* Philadelphia: WB Saunders, 2001. (An advanced reference text for practicing clinicians.)

Maggiore, S.M., L. Brochard. "Pressure-Volume Curve in the Critically Ill." *Curr Opin Crit Care* 2000; 6: 1-10.

Marini, J.J., L. Gattinoni. "Ventilatory Management of Acute Respiratory Distress Syndrome: A Consensus of Two." *Crit Care Med* 2004; 32(1): 250-5.

Pilbeam, S.P., Cairo J.M. *Mechanical Ventilation: Physiological and Clinical Applications.* 4th ed. St. Louis: Mosby, 2006. (A mechanical ventilation teaching text with many examples.)

Takeuchi, M., K.A. Sedeek, G.P. Schettino, K. Suchodolski, R.M. Kacmarek. "Peak Pressure During Volume History and Pressure-Volume Curve Measurement Affects Analysis." *American Journal of Respiratory & Critical Care Medicine* 2001; 164(7):1225-1230.

Tobin, M.J. (ed.). *Principles and Practice of Mechanical Ventilation.* New York: McGraw-Hill, Inc., 1994.

Vieillard-Baron, A., F. Jardin. "The Issue of Dynamic Hyperinflation in Acute Respiratory Distress Syndrome Patients." *European Respiratory Journal* Supplement 2003; 42: 43s-47s.

Walsh, B.K., M.P. Cervinske. "Mechanical Ventilation of the Neonate and Pediatric Patient." In: Cervinske M.P., S.L. Barnhart, editors. *Perinatal and Pediatric Respiratory Care.* Philadelphia: Saunders, 2003: 310-332.

INDEX

M

Maximal expiratory flow rate, 34
Mode, 1

N

Neonatal, 105
  AC pressure control asynchrony,
    117-18
  airleaks, 116
  autocycling, 116
  breath-stacking, 124-25
  control ventilation, 108-9
  cuffless endotracheal tube, 108
  excessive inspiratory pressure
    (beaking), 120
  flow volume loop, 109
  gas exchange, 132
  high frequency ventilation, 132-34
  improper sensitivity setting, 115
  inadequate flow, 119
  infant pulmonary functions, 107
  inspiratory time, 122
  intermittent mandatory ventilation,
    110-111
  large air leak, 116
  lost volume, 108-9
  neonates, 105
  normal scalars, 108
  obstruction to expiratory flow,
    126-27
  pressure control SIMV, 112-13
  pressure limited, 108
  pressure support ventilation,114
  pressure-volume loop, 109
  progression to extubation, 130
  reduced compliance, 121
  respiratory monitoring (benefits), 106
  right mainstem intubation, 128-29
  rise time, 119
  small infants, 105
  termination of inspiratory flow,
    123
  time cycled ventilator, 106
  time triggered, 106
  turbulent baseline flow, 131
Normal scalars, 107

O

Obstruction, 98
Overdistension (beaking), 77, 90

P

Patient triggered breath, 8, 12, 69
Peek expiratory flow rate, 34, 92
Peek flow rate, 47
Peek inspiratory pressure, 2, 6, 10
Plateau pressure, 6, 8, 11
Positive end expiratory pressure
    (PEEP), 28, 87-89
Pressure, 1
Pressure control ventilation (PCV), 20, 51
Pressure limited, 69
Pressure support ventilation (PSV),
    16, 53
Pressure-targeted breath, 41-42, 77-80,
    85
Pressure-targeted controlled
    ventilation, 69
Pressure-volume loop, 1, 23, 53, 69, 108
Pressure vs. time, 1
Pulse oximetry, 18

Q

Quasi-static, 88

R

Rate dyssynchrony, 102
Respiratory frequency (rate), 1-2

S

Scalars, 1
Sensitivity, 101
Sinusoidal (sine) pattern, 35
Spontaneous cycles (breaths), 14, 38
Static compliance, 24
Synchronized intermittent mandatory
    ventilation (SIMV), 8, 14, 53

T

Termination of inspiration, 8
Tidal volume, 1, 10
Time cycled, 69, 77, 85
Transairway pressure, 2, 6

V

Volume cycling, 77, 85
Volume leaks, 103

Volume ventilation, 77-80, 85
Volutrauma, 90